BASIC REHABILITATION TECHNIQUES

A Self-Instructional Guide

Medical Editors

Robert D. Sine, M.D.
Shelly E. Liss, M.D.

Education Editors

Robert E. Roush, Ed.D.
J. David Holcomb, Ed.D.

Assistant Editors

Paul A. Repicky, Ph.D.
Pamela J. Trent, Ph.D.

Contributors

Ruth Avidan, O.T.R.
Marie B, Campbell, R.N.
Joanna B. Chase, M.A.
Leonard E. Heller, Ed.D.
Jane Jester, M.S.W.
Virginia L. Kerr, O.T.R.
Shelly E. Liss, M.D.
Paul A. Repicky, Ph.D.
Robert D. Sine, M.D.
Ruth Stryker-Gordon, R.N., M.A.
Pamela J. Trent, Ph.D.
Georgianna B. Wilson, L.P.T.

BASIC REHABILITATION TECHNIQUES

A Self-Instructional Guide

Edited by

Robert D. Sine, M.D.
Shelly E. Liss, M.D.
Robert E. Roush, Ed.D.
J. David Holcomb, Ed.D.

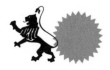

Aspen Systems Corporation
20010 Century Boulevard
Germantown, Maryland
1977

Library of Congress Catalog Card Number: 77-70435
ISBN: 0-912862-38-6

Printed in the United States of America.

1 2 3 4 5

Table of Contents

Preface The Editors vii

Acknowledgements The Editors ix

Prologue *Ruth Stryker-Gordon, R.N., M.A.* xi

Chapter 1 — Common Disability Syndromes 1
Robert D. Sine, M.D.

Chapter 2 — Progressive Mobilization 15
Georgianna B. Wilson, L.P.T.

Chapter 3 — Techniques to Facilitate Communication 109
Joanna B. Chase, M.A., Certified Speech Pathologist

Chapter 4 — Psycho-Social Aspects of Rehabilitation 115
Jane Jester, M.S.W.

Chapter 5 — Self-Care Training for Patients with Hemiplegia, Parkinsonism, and
Arthritis 127
Ruth Avidan, O.T.R.

Chapter 6 — Wheelchairs: Selection, Use, and Maintenance 161
Georgianna Wilson, L.P.T.
Virginia Kerr, O.T.R.

Chapter 7 — Identification and Management of Bowel Problems 175
Robert D. Sine, M.D.

Chapter 8 — Identification and Management of Bladder Problems 181
Shelly E. Liss, M.D.

Chapter 9 — Pressure Sores: Development, Pathogenesis, Prevention, and Treatment 191
Robert D. Sine, M.D.

Chapter 10 — Utilizing Self-Instructional Materials in Rehabilitation Nursing Educa-
tion 203
Paul Repicky, Ph.D.
Pamela Trent, Ph.D.
Leonard Heller, Ed.D.

Epilogue *Marie B. Campbell, R.N.* 215

Contributors' Profiles 217

Index 221

Preface

This book is for all people who, regardless of the cause of their disability, deserve the best care that can be given to them by the practitioners of modern rehabilitation medicine.

The optimal care these patients need is best provided in a facility with a rehabilitation service staffed with a full complement of doctors, nurses, and allied health personnel who have been trained to work together. As a team, these professionals can help restore purpose, function, and dignity to people. Far too often, however, patients suffering from stroke, spinal cord injury, or other degenerative diseases languish in hospitals and long term care facilities. General duty nurses are thus placed in the position of attempting to devise care plans by themselves that actually require the specialist training of five or six other health professionals. Unfortunately, this is the rule, not the exception.

The Editors are confident that any health professional with patient care responsibilities can learn something from this book which will be valuable to them and to their patients. But it is mainly for nurses that this book has been written, because the nurse is still the common denominator in translating the physician's orders into action at the bedside. The nurse is often the patient's only hope of receiving compassion and encouragement. The nurse, in the absence of other rehabilitation personnel, must alone take care of patients whose bodies require restoration and whose perceptions of personal worth must be maintained.

Through grants from the Regional Medical Program of Texas to Rosewood General Hospital and Baylor College of Medicine, a training manual and a series of workshops were designed to improve the quality of rehabilitative nursing care. For three years, nurses with inservice education responsibilities from primarily small, rural hospitals used the manuals at Rosewood in workshops conducted under the aegis of the Center for Allied Health Manpower Development at Baylor College of Medicine. After completing the educational program, the nurse-trainees were able to return home and teach others the new techniques they had learned.

This book was conceived because of the relationship stemming from workshop collaboration between hospital staff and medical school faculty. Thus, the contents of this book have been thoroughly tested by time in the clinical setting and evaluated in the trainees' home hospitals following the workshops they attended in Houston. We hope you, the readers, will appreciate the nursing input to this effort as much as we have. We also hope that you sense the spirit of the camaraderie of team care that characterizes this book.

The Editors
Houston, Texas
June 1977

Acknowledgements

A book would not be a book without the help of many other people. This one is no exception. It has been a team effort in the best rehabilitation tradition. The contributors were the same people who pulled together on the ward every day. Professionals in the purest sense of the word, they wrote on their own time for an audience expected to be small, but important. Without their contributions, the original training grant and this book would not have been possible. Although Georgianna Wilson's contribution as an author has been recognized, we owe her a special debt of gratitude inasmuch as she not only helped run the many workshops held at Rosewood but also greatly assisted us in the preparation of this final draft. Her efforts were indispensable.

Those not listed as contributors, but to whom we also want to express our gratitude are:

- Linda Arfele, R.N., who reviewed several sections of this book from her point of view as a working rehabilitation nurse;
- Beulah Waltmon, who was perhaps the most important person to the overall project since she typed the entire book at least six times from longhand manuscripts that ranged in legibility from zero to at best a five on a ten-point scale; and
- Dr. Gerald Hirschberg, whose ingenious exercise program was of such central importance it is doubtful that we could have begun without it.

The Editors also want to recognize the vital roles played by Rosewood General Hospital and Baylor College of Medicine. In the final analysis, it was the cooperation between the administrative staff in both institutions that allowed the workshops to be held and, consequently, the book to be written.

In closing, we want to thank two distinguished nurses for having written the Prologue and Epilogue for us. Ruth Stryker-Gordon, the author of several books on rehabilitation nursing, sets the stage for the book in the Prologue. Marie Campbell, the head nurse of a rehabilitation unit, summarizes the purpose of the book in the Epilogue.

The Editors
Houston, Texas
June 1977

Prologue

Rehabilitation is both a simple and a complex component of nursing. It is simple because the necessary knowledge and skills are relatively uncomplicated. It is complex because these relatively uncomplicated skills draw from a variety of disciplines; namely, medicine, physical therapy, occupational therapy, speech therapy, and social work, as well as basic nursing. For the severely disabled, a team of health professionals is needed for initial care. For the less severely disabled and for the continued care of all disabled persons, the nurse can attend to the majority of patient needs and refer special problems to the appropriate professional.

It is tragic that some physicians, nurses, and other health professionals are unfamiliar with the dramatic outcomes of both preventive and therapeutic rehabilitative measures. Lack of this awareness often keeps the patient from care that is available. In addition, iatrogenic and "nursigenic" conditions—those caused by both the commission of inappropriate care and omission of care—develop in already disabled persons, making it necessary for rehabilitation teams to deal with the person's disability and preventable conditions.

This book recognizes these problems. Its content has been developed from the salient contribution that each health profession makes to rehabilitation. Each section of the book has been developed by the specialist who can best contribute to that content being addressed.

The self-instructional aspect of this book gives nurses an opportunity to check their understanding of concepts and skills throughout. It also enables nurses to go at their own pace—slow, fast, interrupted, review, whatever. Once a nurse masters these techniques, the final test, of course, remains: Will he or she apply them when the person with a stroke, spinal cord injury, arthritis, fracture, or Parkinsonism is admitted for care? If you are one who does, you will assist disabled persons to regain optimum functions in minimal time. If you forget, you could cause undue hospitalization, unnecessary expense, preventable complications, and unwarranted periods of discouragement and frustration.

Because most practicing nurses do not see their patients long enough to see such outcomes, they could be oblivious to them. The authors of this book hope that its readers will be attuned to the positive effects of the application of these rehabilitation techniques. Our patients will be the ones to gain in mobility, morale, and function. What else could give greater satisfaction to a practicing nurse in any setting? I know of none.

Ruth Stryker-Gordon, R.N., M.A.

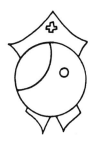

Common Disability Syndromes

ROBERT D. SINE, M.D.

1.

Introduction and Objectives

We have coined the phrase "disability syndrome" for two reasons: (1) to enable us to discuss in a reasonable space a common constellation of disabilities despite multiple etiologies; (2) to emphasize that a common therapeutic approach to these disabilities is workable. If you can recognize a portion of a syndrome, you can begin an evaluation by examining for the presence of the associated disabilities. You can then proceed to utilize specific therapy for the disabilities whether the original insult was vascular, tumor, or any other of the many possibilities. Upon completion of this chapter, you should be able to:

1. discuss the rehabilitation problems of patients with hemiplegia, spinal cord dysfunction, Parkinsonism, and arthritis;
2. identify the causes of common disability problems; and
3. identify some selected treatments for disability problems.

Disability Syndrome of Hemiplegia

Most of us, on a day-to-day basis, find the disability most frequently encountered is hemiplegia. This is to be expected since as of 1961 there were an estimated 1.8 million living hemiparetic Americans. The figure is undoubtedly higher today. So much contact leads to familiarity and the assumption that we "know" the syndrome. The syndrome is complex, however. It occurs with injury to the sensorimotor cortex and its pathways. These are the intricate structures whose functions raise man beyond the other mammals. The effects of their impairment cannot be simple.

Anatomy

The sensorimotor cortex lies along the upper middle surface of the hemisphere (Figure 1-1). The neurons in this area send forth axons, which converge deeper within the hemisphere where they can be seen as an L-shaped area of white tissue known as the internal capsule (early anatomists thought it was

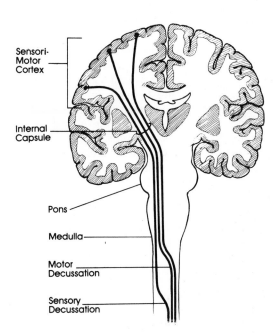

Sensori-
Motor
Cortex

Internal
Capsule

Pons

Medulla

Motor
Decussation

Sensory
Decussation

Figure 1-1   Frontal Cross Section of the Brain

a capsule). Beyond the internal capsule the fibers continue through the pons to the medulla, where first the sensory then the motor axons cross to the opposite side (decussate). It is the decussation that decides that the right side of the brain will control the left side of the body, and the left side of the brain the right side of the body.

Pathophysiology

Any agent that attacks the sensorimotor cortex or its pathways can produce the hemiparetic syndrome. Included in the many possible lesions are direct trauma and trauma productive of subdural hematoma; benign tumor; malignant primary, and metastatic tumor; abscess, arterio-venous malformation, hemorrhage, and infarction.

Tissue death secondary to loss of its blood supply (infarction) is the most common cause of the syndrome. It is well known that, with aging, atherosclerosis progressively destroys the competence of the arteries. The final events preceding tissue death are less well defined, however. Present opinion known as the "embolic" theory holds that the final chain of events begins with ulceration of the atherosclerotic plaque, and clot formation on its surface. Plaque and/or clot fragments then embolize to lodge in more distal arteries. Eventually the original clot may form a thrombus large enough to occlude the artery (Figure 1-2). The importance of the theory is that it suggests some practical possibilities for prophylaxis.

The emboli can give rise to neurological symptoms diagnosed as transient ischemic attacks (TIAs). These are considered as a tip-off that a large irreversible episode of infarction is imminent. A work-up including angiography frequently demonstrates that the origin of the emboli is in an artery accessible to surgical repair.[1]

Hemispheric Specialization

It is said that each hemisphere "specializes." The most obvious example of a specialized function is that of speech, which resides in the left hemisphere. When the left hemisphere is damaged, as in right hemiplegia, speech functions are usually impaired (aphasia). More subtle forms of

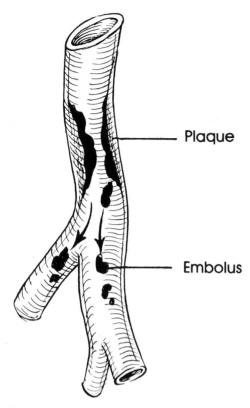

Plaque

Embolus

Figure 1-2

specialization are only recently being discovered.[2,3,4]

Table 1-1 is a partial listing of functions concentrated in one hemisphere. Note that the faculties under "ideation" are ways of thinking or contrasting approaches to problem solving. It might be helpful to think of two "personalities" within each of us, each offering its own complementary approach to our problems. In hemiplegia, when one hemisphere is injured, the "personality" of the intact hemisphere becomes dominant. Sequential ideation can be overheard in most therapy departments as the left hemiplegic patient rehearses ambulation: "*One*: lift foot. *Two*: bend knee. *Three*: swing foot," etc. You can also observe right hemiplegics using their special forms of ideation to pick up difficult ADL (activities of daily living) tasks despite complete lack of understanding of spoken instruction. It has been observed that patients with left hemiplegia tend to deny or belittle their failures. In contrast, right hemiplegics react to failure with increased anxiety. Left hemiplegics learn faster but have more difficulty with retention.

Despite this right-left specialization, there is a great deal of overlap. The functions we call "mind"—behavior, personality, intellect, memory, emotion—reside in the cortical hemispheres: yet it is possible to completely remove either hemisphere with little disturbance of these functions. This information suggests two major points to be made which are important to the teaching of rehabilitation skills:

1. There is enough overlap of functions between the hemispheres that a patient with either hemisphere intact can be taught complex skills despite extensive damage of the other hemisphere.
2. We must tailor our methods of teaching to the residual capacities in the undamaged hemisphere.

In practical terms, the most obvious example is the case of an aphasic patient. He will get little from spoken instruction but could grasp a skill such as putting on a shirt quickly if it is presented in pantomime. A more subtle example is that of the left hemiplegic who might learn the skill more easily if it is broken into short steps presented in a linear fashion.

We must evaluate first—then teach. An input inappropriate to the patient's intact senses is as useless to the hemiplegic as providing books to the blind or records to the deaf. This might tax the ingenuity of the nurse-teacher but offers renewed hope for success. The full capacities for learning lie in each hemisphere if we will but use both of our hemispheres to approach the patient's remaining hemisphere on its own ground.

Paresis—Its Distribution and Clinical Course

The distribution of weakness tends to follow a "typical" pattern of severity in hemiplegia. The leg generally retains more strength than the arm. The leg extensors, which straighten the leg, return earlier and remain stronger than the flexors. This is fortunate as these are the muscles of primary concern in standing and walking.

By contrast, in the upper extremity the flexors dominate.[5] Functional use of the upper extremity requires fine coordination of the shoulder to enable hand placement in addition to a prehensile hand. It is instructive to note a functional upper extremity is seldom regained if it is not present by the third month following onset.[6] It is all too common an experience to find a massive therapeutic investment in the paretic hand, destined to be futile, while the critical skills for the "well" arm, as described in Chapter 5, have been ignored.

The pattern of returning reflexes, strength, and other phenomena is referred to by clinicians as spontaneous neurological return. Recent evidence suggests there could be peripheral as well as central neurophysiology responsible for the observed changes.[7,8] There is no evidence to suggest, however, that any therapeutic efforts available alter this physiological process.

If you are working with hemiplegia secondary to cerebral thrombosis, you can look forward to a degree of this type of return. As it occurs, every use should be made of it; but you must guard against perpetuating useless therapeutics on the belief they were responsible for the natural event.

Spasticity

The contraction of a "spastic" muscle is set off by the same reflexes that jerk your knee when the tendon is tapped with a percussion hammer. In the patient with spasticity these reflexes are exaggerated because of loss of their control by neurons in the brain. The reflexes are set off by sensors ("muscle spindles") in the muscle which respond to *acceleration* of stretch.[9] This is why you can often stretch a muscle slowly without it "fighting" you, but an attempt to do it faster is futile (see Chapter 2). We have found Dantrium to be very helpful in relieving spasticity present in selected hemiparetic patients. This drug is thought to act peripherally.[10] On a short term basis the side effect of weakness has been a limitation. Long term, the possibility of liver damage may preclude use in young patients. The dosage must be titrated carefully to achieve the desired effect of minimum spasticity and maximum strength.

Sensory Loss

Loss of sensation can vary widely in the hemiplegic patient. Occasionally it can be so severe in the upper extremity that the patient can mangle his hand in the wheelchair spokes without being aware of it. In the leg the loss most likely to produce difficulty is loss of position sense. Severe loss of this modality in the knee can produce instability when standing on it despite adequate strength. Retraining is very effective in regaining function despite persistent sensory deficit.

TABLE 1-1
Hemispheric Specialization

| The right side of the brain has (the right hemiplegic retains; the left hemiplegic has lost) | Motor control of (L) side of body. Sensation from the (L) side of the body. Sight from the (L) visual fields. Timbre (musical). Ideation which is: visual-spectral, gestalt-synesthetic, and has a tendency for creativity. | The left side of the brain has (the left hemiplegic retains; the right hemiplegic has lost) | Motor control of (R) side of body. Sensation from the (R) side of the body. Language faculties: (symbol use) use and understanding of speech and writing and reading. Arithmetical ability. Ideation which is: analytical-propositional-logical and linear in time (sequential). |

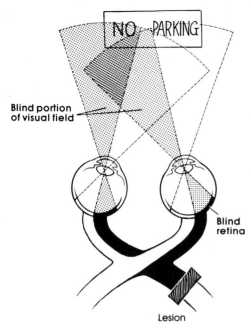

Figure 1-3

Sight lost on the side of the hemiplegia shifts as the center of attention shifts.

Homonymous Hemianopia

Homonymous hemianopia is the loss of half of the visual field on the same side of each eye. It commonly appears with hemiplegia and results in blindness on the same side of the hemiplegia. This can occur because only one-half of the optic fibers decussate. Figure 1-3 is a schematic of how the tracts from each side of the brain go to the retina on the same side of each eye.

This type of blindness is a much more serious problem than is generally realized. It is much more disabling than one-eye blindness. You may suppose that all a person with left homonymous hemianopia need do when, for example, he reads a sign would be to look slightly to the left thus encompassing the whole of the sign within his remaining right visual field. In practice, however, mechanisms in the brain "lock in" the eyes so that the point of our attention is at the center of the visual fields. The patient therefore only sees half of whatever he looks at (see Figure 1-3).

When severe, the disability can be considerable. A "No Parking" sign could be read "Parking." He might eat from only one side of his plate, write only on one side of the page, and clothe only the intact side of his body. Training to compensate for this loss is difficult, but possible and most essential (see Chapter 5).

Verticality Perception

Often a hemiparetic patient can be observed sitting with a lean to his hemiparetic side. A suggestion to sit straight will sometimes produce a position even further from the vertical. An attempt to stand puts the patient in danger of falling to that side. Often this is the major barrier to transfers and ambulation. Experiments have demonstrated that this is a perceptual deficit that can be measured by asking the patient to report the verticality of a luminous rod in a darkened room.[11,12] The patient "sees" the world on a slant (Figure 1-4). The balance training described in Chapter 2 is directed at compensating for the effects of this damaging phenomenon and is often a prerequisite for ambulation.

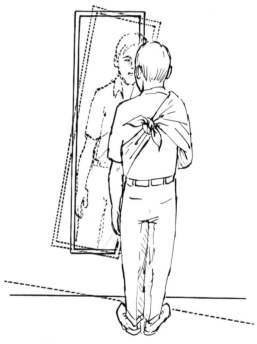

Figure 1-4

The world is seen rotated to the side of the hemiplegia.

Posttest for Hemiplegia

Let's see how much you have learned. Select the correct answer to complete the following statements.

1. In utilizing rehabilitation techniques:
   a. You should begin with the most challenging activity.
   b. You should assure the patient that with a little work he will be normal.
   c. You should not begin until the diagnosis has been established.
   d. You may proceed with disability-specific therapy even if the diagnosis is not known.

2. The brain:
   a. Works like a marvelous perfectly efficient computer.
   b. Is organized so each piece of knowledge is stored in a particular place.
   c. Is organized so that each hemisphere has different but overlapping functions.
   d. Uses very little energy.

3. Hemiplegia (weakness at one side of the body):
   a. Is synonymous with cerebral vascular accident.
   b. Is produced only by a lesion in the internal capsule.
   c. Usually present in concert with other disabilities.
   d. All the above.

4. Cerebral infarction:
   a. Is the death of cerebral tissue secondary to insufficient blood flow.
   b. Occurs when cerebral arteries are blocked by thrombi.
   c. Occurs when cerebral arteries are blocked by emboli.
   d. All the above.

5. A patient with right hemiplegia:
   a. Has a lesion on the right side of his brain.
   b. Has a right visual field defect.
   c. Has serious impairment of visuo-spatial perception.
   d. None of the above.

6. A patient who sits leaning to his hemiplegic side:
   a. Will walk just as easily as one who sits upright.
   b. Only needs to be reminded to sit up straight.
   c. Probably does so because of weak trunk muscles.
   d. Can benefit from balance training.
   e. All the above.

7. The visual field defect of hemiplegia:
   a. Is called a homonymous hemianopia.
   b. Can be very disabling.
   c. Is on the side of the hemiplegia.
   d. All the above.

8. Right and left hemiplegic disability syndromes:
   a. Are simply mirror images of each other.
   b. Are differentiated mainly by the right hemiplegic's aphasia.
   c. Are differentiated mainly by the left hemiplegic's retention of the dominant hand.
   d. Are differentiated by a large number of "higher" brain functions.

9. The left hemisphere:
   a. Is intact in the right hemiplegic.
   b. Solves problems in a linear fashion.
   c. Enables us to draw hexagons.
   d. Is larger and visibly more complex than the right hemisphere.

10. Spasticity:
    a. Produces massive jerks which may throw the hemiplegic to the floor.
    b. Is relieved by any good "muscle relaxor."
    c. Is produced by uninhibited stretch reflexes.
    d. Is painful.

11. The hemiplegic secondary to cerebrovascular accident typically:
    a. Has a "fixed" lesion: he neither improves nor gets worse.
    b. Can expect some neurologic improvement with or without treatment.
    c. Can expect some neurologic improvement with vasodilators.
    d. Can expect some neurologic improvements with Vitamin B12.
    e. Can expect some neurologic improvements with physical therapy.

The correct answers are as follows:

1.	d	7.	d
2.	c	8.	d
3.	c	9.	b
4.	d	10.	c
5.	b	11.	b
6.	d		

If you missed any of the questions, you should review that section of this chapter.

Disability Syndrome of Spinal Cord Dysfunction

The patient with spinal cord dysfunction demands our attention as much because of functions he is spared as those he has lost. He is left with a clear mind and a normal life span. Small wonder he uses both to push us to help minimize his devastating losses and question their permanence.

The extent of the loss is directly related to the level of the injury and whether it is "complete" or "partial." A complete lesion is one which stops all neural transmission at the level of the lesion. "Partial" lesions can range from minimal deficits to those just short of complete. Unfortunately, because the spinal cord is a narrow structure, the majority of lesions are complete.

Table 1-2 is an attempt to show the disability incurred at crucial levels of injury. Study it carefully and refer to it when you have patients with such injuries. Remember that at each level the patient suffers all the disabilities that occur at the lower (caudal) levels as well as those at that particular level. Thus all complete lesions will have loss of control of the bowel, bladder, and sexual organs. A C_5 lesion will have those disabilities listed and, in addition, all those listed below it. It is also important to know that spasticity occurs below the injured level. Both Valium and Dantrium have been helpful in managing the spasticity.

You will note that while an athletic and determined patient may manage a form of ambulation at high levels, past L_4 most ambulation is the high energy cost "swing-through"

type (see Chapter 2), and this becomes increasingly less functional as trunk stability is lost. Preoccupation with ambulation that is less efficient than wheelchair use occasionally leads to lower overall functional capacity. You will also note the drastic deterioration of hand functions with each lost cervical segment. The lost prehension and residual wrist extension peculiar to injury at the sixth cervical level allows the use of assistive devices designed to harness wrist extension to move the fingers for prehension (see Figure 1-5). Many of the more general assistive devices described in Chapter 5 might be found to have a place as well. Patients with the high lesions (above C_7) may find externally powered devices helpful, but to date these have found limited acceptance. One probably crucial reason is that these patients usually require full time assistants if they are to be cared for outside of an institution. High lesions could have respiratory problems because of paralysis of the intercostals. Patients who survive injuries as high as C_3 require continuous assistance with

TABLE 1-2
Spinal Cord Disability Syndrome

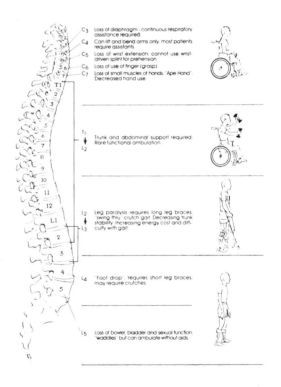

C_3	Loss of diaphragm - continuous respiratory assistance required.
C_4	Can lift and bend arms only, most patients require assistants.
C_5	Loss of wrist extension, cannot use wrist-driven splint for prehension.
C_6	Loss of use of finger (grasp).
C_7	Loss of small muscles of hands, "Ape Hand". Decreased hand use.
T_1 – L_2	Trunk and abdominal support required. Rare functional ambulation.
L_2 – L_3	Leg paralysis requires long leg braces, "swing thru" crutch gait. Decreasing trunk stability. Increasing energy cost and difficulty with gait.
L_4	"Foot drop", requires short leg braces, may require crutches.
L_5	Loss of bowel, bladder and sexual function. "Waddles" but can ambulate without aids.

respiration because of paralysis of the diaphragm.

Of course, since all sensation and movement is lost below the injured level, these patients are among the most vulnerable to decubiti. The chapters on decubiti, bowel, bladder, and social service will all be of interest if you are attending a patient with spinal cord dysfunction at any level.

Sex is always discussed last in this type of essay, but the subject has not wanted for attention in recent years. Writers advocate varying therapy, but all suggest open discussion and experimentation.[13] Sensation is lost; but erection is frequently possible and male fertility also possible, though of diminished likelihood. Women require artifical lubrication but suffer no reduction of fertility.

Posttest for Spinal Cord Dysfunction

Select the correct answer to complete the following statements:

1. *A patient with a complete lesion at spinal cord level L_4, retains:*
   a. *Sexual function.*
   b. *Bowel and bladder control.*
   c. *Lower extremity function.*
   d. *Trunk stability.*
2. *The paraplegic has no difficulty with:*
   a. *Ambulation.*
   b. *Spasticity.*
   c. *Intellectual loss.*
   d. *Bladder control.*
3. *Paraplegic ambulation:*
   a. *Becomes progressively less functional the higher the level of the lesion.*
   b. *Should not overwhelm other considerations, which ultimately could be more important.*
   c. *Requires long leg braces at the L_3 and above levels.*
   d. *All the above.*

Compare your answers to the following correct answers:

   1. *d*
   2. *c*
   3. *d*

If you missed any of the questions, please review that section of the chapter before proceeding.

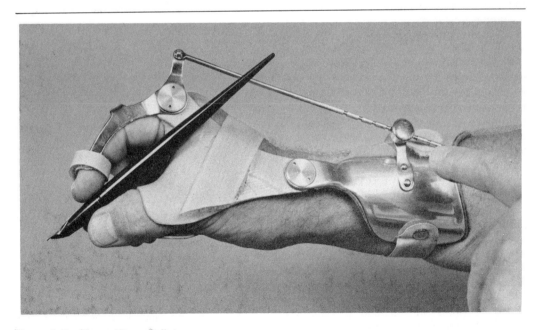

Figure 1-5 Flexor Hinge Splint

(Courtesy of T.J. Engen, Orthotist.)

Disability Syndrome of Parkinsonism

The disabilities of Parkinsonism are so widespread, yet so poorly understood, that we often think of them as just part of getting old. Young actors who play old people assume an expressionless face, speak with a strained monotonal voice, and affect a hand tremor and shuffling gait. They are unaware that they are not portraying age but the symptoms of a disease. When an old man is quite free of Parkinson symptomatology we say he's "spry," designating the absence rather than the presence of disease. The onset of symptoms is very slow and insidious. Though they are not disabling in their early stages, they do cut down the patient's mobility and safety. It is likely many a broken hip is a complication of early Parkinsonism. One may argue whether it is the insidious onset or a sad reflection of our disinterest in the elderly which produces the general complacency surrounding this syndrome. It is a fact, however, that the symptoms are frequently untreated.

This seems particularly true of patients who lack the characteristic "pill-rolling" tremor of the hands. These patients may still have the syndrome's most disabling symptoms. These result from a slowness in initiating movement. The patient may have great difficulty arising from a chair. His muscles may be strong but he has difficulty initiating the movement. Once standing he could have difficulty initiating corrective movements if he starts to fall. He might complain of "bad balance"—do not be surprised if he is on drugs for vertigo. You can test such a patient by giving him a gentle push on the chest backward. He will tend to fall like a piece of timber; have a hand at his back to catch him. You might also note on observing his gait that he has difficulty starting, stopping, and turning. There is nothing wrong with his muscles of deglutition, but if he does not swallow spontaneously, saliva collects in his mouth and he will drool. He might also seem dull; his face is expressionless, and his verbal responses are often delayed. It is all too natural to forget that his mind is quite clear and talk around or through him.

Another phenomenon—rigidity—may be present. Rigidity is never so severe that the muscles cannot be stretched and the joint cannot be put through range of motion. Rigidity plus the paucity of movement, however, may lead to contractures. The severely involved patient with multiple contractures requiring total bed care, but with a clear mind, is the other end of the Parkinsonism spectrum. Unfortunately this patient often goes untreated as does the early patient, for he is supposed beyond help. The supposition becomes a self-fulfilling prophesy.

The Parkinsonism syndrome is produced when structures deep within the brain—the basal ganglia—are damaged. In the majority of cases the mechanism is unknown. The syndrome may rarely occur following encephalitis. Recent work with monkeys[14] indicates that volitional activity initiates in the basal ganglia, making these structures a higher center for motor control than the motor cortex. This information suggests an explanation for some of the phenomena observed in Parkinsonism.

Much of the material in later chapters will deal with motor activities. When dealing with Parkinsonism patients it will be well to recall the peculiar features of slowness in initating a change in movement patterns. In practical terms this means: (1) you must allow for a long "reaction time" while giving instructions; (2) the patient must develop "start up" techniques; (3) the early patient could have selective difficulty with specific activities (turning, getting up from a chair); (4) the severely involved patient could have more potential than is evident from superficial observation.

Undoubtedly, the most significant advance in treatment has been the use of L-dopa for relief of symptoms. This drug has preempted the use of earlier anti-Parkinsonism compounds in our practice. We are convinced the addition of a compound (inhibitor) preventing breakdown of the L-dopa peripherally facilitates administration. A useful combination drug is available (Sinemet®), which seems to enhance overall effectiveness.

Vitamin B_6 can reverse the effects of the drug. The B-complex vitamins are known as "good for nerves," and as patients are often secretive regarding self-medication, the nurse is often in a better position than the physician to discover if any antagonistic drugs are being taken.

Techniques described in the following chapters can make significant differences in the quality of life of patients with Parkinsonism, although it is true that the wide prevalence of this disease makes it something of an overwhelming problem that is hardly an excuse for neglecting the individual. Rewards can still be gratifying, dealing as we must, with a patient at a time.

Posttest for Parkinsonism

Select the correct answer:

1. *Symptoms of Parkinsonism do not include:*
   a. *Rigidity.*
   b. *Shuffling gait.*
   c. *Spasticity.*
   d. *Hand tremor.*
2. *Drugs of value in treating Parkinsonism are:*
   a. *L-dopa.*
   b. *Valium.*
   c. *Vitamin B_6.*
   d. *Dantrium.*
3. *The lesion producing Parkinsonism is in the:*
   a. *Internal capsule.*
   b. *Cerebral cortex.*
   c. *Basal ganglia.*
   d. *Muscles.*

The correct answers are as follows:
1. *c*   2. *a*   3. *c*

Check your answers. If you missed any, you should review that section of this chapter.

Disability Syndrome of Arthritis

Disease of the joints is so widespread it is easy to forget that the "pain and stiffness of arthritis" can constitute serious disabilities. There are numerous diseases which may affect the joints, but by far the most important are osteoarthritis and rheumatoid arthritis.

Rheumatoid Arthritis

Rheumatoid arthritis starts in the lining of the joint (the synovium). It tends to be very destructive and may attack the underlying cartilage and bone as well. An acutely involved joint is warm, swollen, and red. Deformity of the joint is accelerated by the swelling, which loosens the ligaments that hold the bones forming the joint in position. The laxity at the joint produced by the swelling allows the bones to slip out of their normal position (subluxate). This usually occurs in the direction of strongest use. In the hand this mechanism may produce subluxation at the wrist and metacarpophalangeal joints (Figure 1-6). You can see how in this stage (when joints are swollen) use of the hand could promote deformity.

With time the structures surrounding the joint become tight and the deformities become fixed. When attempting to correct these deformities by stretching the joint, linear pull should be exerted (Figure 1-6). An episode would follow this sequence:

1. Appearance of warm, swollen, painful joint.
2. Joint subluxation (slippage).
3. Periarticular structures tighten, "fixing" the deformity in its new, deformed position.

Management

Commonly, the patient with arthritis is told he needs "rest and exercise." This sounds contradictory, but it is not since at every stage both rest and exercise are necessary. The proper balance is determined by the degree of inflammatory response: the more inflammation, the more rest and less exercise; and vice versa. In the acute stage, movement of the joint is painful and additionally aggravates the inflammation. The episode is shortened if both the joint and the patient are rested as much as possible. In this stage the "rest" half of the "rest and exercise" prescription is most important. Splints are occasionally used to ensure resting the joint. "Exercise" is usually only a few movements carefully done through the range of motion to the point of pain. That ensures retention of mobility. Suspension of the joint in warm water could make these maneuvers less painful and more complete.

You will know the inflammation is decreasing as the joint swelling and warmth subside

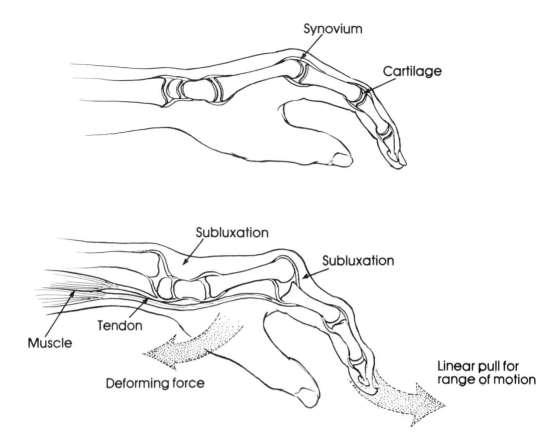

Synovium

Cartilage

Subluxation

Subluxation

Muscle

Tendon

Deforming force

Linear pull for range of motion

Figure 1-6 Common Disability Syndromes

and pain lessens. Then range of motion exercises can be more vigorous in that they should be encouraged in the face of discomfort. Vigorous use of the joint should be resumed only after active inflammation is judged to be absent.

Then the patient may also engage in the full spectrum of an active life. In this disease, however, there should be no pressure to engage in exercise for its own sake or the impression that it will "cure" the disease. Most patients are subject to episodes of recurrence. With these cautions in mind, the mobilization program and activities of daily living chapters in this book may be applied. Exercise should have increased function as its goal, and energy conservation techniques and assistive devices should be utilized as they are found helpful.

Aspirin is still the mainstay of drug therapy. Unfortunately the public holds this familiar drug in ill-deserved contempt. This is probably because they are familiar only with its analgesic properties. One of the most valuable services nursing personnel can perform is educating the patient in the value of aspirin for its antiinflammatory effect and the need to adhere to prescribed dosage schedules (on the order of twelve tablets per day) to obtain that effect. Motrin, Indomethecin, gold salts, antimalarials, and oral corticosteroids all have their place in drug therapy for rheumatoid arthritis. In each case, however, the beneficial effects must be carefully weighed against side effects. Intra-articular corticosteroids are very helpful in aborting an acute attack or remobilizing one or two joints; it cannot be used with multiple joint involvement.

Osteoarthritis

Osteoarthritis starts with degeneration of the cartilage. Replacement of the degenerated cartilage by bone and subsequent overgrowth of the bone produces the deformity of bony enlargement of the joints. The joints affected are largely weight-bearing joints such as the knees, hips, and joints of the spine. The exceptions to this rule are the small joints of the fingers. The condition progresses slowly, and despite being very prevalent in the population seldom causes disability before the fifth decade. By the age of seventy, however, few individuals are entirely free of it; and significant numbers of disabled individuals—mostly from hip involvement—are seen at sixty years old and older.

The first lines of defense for hip involvement are proper use of a cane and range of motion exercises (see Chapter 2). Use of the cane can unweight the hip 80 percent.[14] You must emphasize to the cane-user that:

1. he will not become "dependent" on the cane, and muscles will not atrophy;
2. he will slow the disease and prolong the useful life of the hip; and
3. he will be able to walk further, see and do more, and lead a fuller life with its use.

Intra-articular corticosteroid injection has been helpful to gain range of motion in the hip and control acute episodes in the knee. Involvement of the fingers is seldom disabling (except for specific activities such as typing) but can be painful and can produce unattractive deformity. Heat applied by water or paraffin helps relieve the pain.

Aspirin is also valuable in management of osteoarthritis. Butazolidine and Indomethecine have been used particularly for hip involvement. Total hip replacement has been the most successful surgical approach.

A comparison of rheumatoid arthritis and osteoarthritis is summarized in Table 1-3.

Posttest for Arthritis

Select the correct answers to complete the following statements:

1. *The primary site of involvement in the joint of rheumatoid arthritis is:*
   a. *The cartilage.*
   b. *The bone.*
   c. *The endothelium.*
   d. *The synovium.*
2. *Osteoarthritis:*
   a. *Is a disease of the ends of the bones.*
   b. *Produces red hot swollen joints.*
   c. *Is very prevalent in the geriatric population.*
   d. *Has a rapid downhill course and disablement in 2 years.*
3. *Intra-articular corticosteroids:*
   a. *Can be helpful in managing osteoarthritis.*
   b. *Can be helpful in managing rheumatoid arthritis.*
   c. *Can be helpful in joint remobilization.*
   d. *All the above.*
   e. *(b) and (c) only.*

TABLE 1-3
Comparison of Rheumatoid Arthritis and Osteoarthritis

Factor	Rheumatoid Arthritis	Osteoarthritis
Primary tissue involvement	Synovium	Cartilage
Type of disease	"Systemic"—connective tissue throughout body involved	Degenerative local "wear and tear"
Joints (location)	Any synovial joint	Weight-bearing joints (hips, knees, spine) and fingers
Joints (appearance)	Spindle-shaped, soft swelling, symmetrical	"Knobby" enlarged joints
Blood	Positive latex fixation test; increased sedimentation rate	No blood changes
Course	Acute severe episodes of synovial swelling and warmth. Can produce joint destruction and deformity	Slow-boney enlargement produces large, boney joints and limitation of range of motion

4. "*Rest and exercise*" in managing rheumatoid arthritis means:
   a. There should be a period of rest after each exercise period.
   b. Different types and amounts of each depending on the extent of inflammatory activity.
   c. As much exercise as possible and then a rest period.
   d. "Rest" is for the joint—not the patient.
   e. "Rest" is for the patient—not the joint.

The correct answers are as follows:

1. *d*
2. *c*
3. *d*
4. *b*

If you missed any of the questions, please review the section on arthritis.

Notes

1. W. Field, *"Clinical Symposia," CIBA* 26 (1974): 3-31.
2. J.E. Bogen, "The Other Side of the Brain I: Dysgraphia and Dycopia Following Cerebral Commissurotomy," *Los Angeles Neurological Societies Bulletin* 34 (April 1969): 73-105.
3. J.E. Bogen, "The Other Side of the Brain II: An Oppositional Mind," *Los Angeles Neurological Societies Bulletin* 34 (July 1969): 135-169.
4. J.E. Bogen and G.M. Bogen, "The Other Side of the Brain III: The Corpus Collosium and Creativity," *Los Angeles Neurological Societies Bulletin* 37 (1972): 49-61.
5. T.E. Twitchell, "The Restoration of Motor Function in Hemiplegia," *Neurology* 4 (December 1954): 919-928.
6. G. Bard and G. Hirshberg, "Recovery of Voluntary Motion in Upper Extremity Following Hemiplegia," *Archives of Physical Medicine and Rehabilitation* 46 (August 1965): 567-575.
7. O. Goldkamp, "Electromyography and Nerve Conduction Studies in 116 Patients with Hemiplegia," *Archives of Physical Medicine and Rehabilitation* 98 (February 1957): 59-63.
8. E. Johnson, "Sequence of Electromyographic Abnormalities in Stroke Syndrome," *Archives of Physical Medicine and Rehabilitation* 56 (November 1975).
9. R. Herman, "Myotatic Reflex: Clinico-Physiological Aspects of Spasticity and Contracture," *Brain* 93 (1970): 273-312.
10. A.W. Monster, "Spasticity and the Effect of Dantrulene Sodium," *Archives of Physical Medicine and Rehabilitation* 55 (August 1974): 363-383.
11. D. De Censio, "Vertical Perception and Ambulation in Hemiplegia," *Archives of Physical Medicine and Rehabilitation* 51 (February 1970): 105-110.
12. J.H. Bruell, "Disturbance of Perception of Verticality in Patients with Hemiplegia," *Archives of Physical Medicine and Rehabilitation* 38 (December 1957): 776-780.
13. E.W. Everts, "Brain Mechanism in Movement," *Scientific American* 229 (July 1973): 96-103.

Suggested Readings

Alphers, B.J. *Clinical Neurology.* Philadelphia: F.A. Davis Co., 1963.

Blount, W. "Don't Throw Away the Cane." *Journal of Bone and Joint Surgery* 38-A (June 1956): 695-708.

Bogen, J.E. "Introduction to Hemipherectomy." In *Drugs, Development and Cerebral Function.* Smith, W.L., editor. Springfield, Illinois: Charles C. Thomas, 1971.

Cerebrovascular Study Group Survey Report. Bethesda, Md.: Institute of Neurological Diseases and Blindness, National Institutes of Health, 1961.

Diller, L. "Brain Damage and Rehabilitation." In *Neuropsychology of Spatially-Oriented Behavior.* Freedman, S.F., editor. Homewood, Illinois: Dorsey Press, 1968.

Fordyce, W.E., and Jones, R.H. "Efficacy of Oral and Pantomine Instructions for Hemiplegic Patients." *Archives of Physical Medicine and Rehabilitation 47 (October 1966): 676-680.*

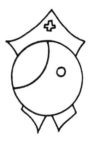

Progressive Mobilization

Georgianna Wilson, L.P.T.

2.

Introduction

You may be wondering what "Progressive Mobilization" is. Let me put your mind at ease. In completing this chapter you will learn techniques for the gradual, step-by-step development of a patient's ability to move around. The activities discussed start with the patient lying in bed and end with the patient up and walking.

Due to the amount of material in this chapter we have divided it into 4 sections. These sections are interrelated and arranged sequentially. You may use any one unit independently, but to make effective use of the Progressive Mobilization Program, you must understand the relationships among these units. The importance of these relationships is demonstrated through the use of a "staircase" model to progressive mobilization. You will learn that if you decide to use the techniques in the last section with a patient, the steps in the preceding sections must have been completed.

The intent in writing and selecting the material for this chapter is that it be information *necessary* to rehabilitate your patient. For example, the discussion of normal gait brings out points pertinent to the activities being taught and is not a comprehensive discussion of the subject. Other areas are discussed in the same manner. The material is *basic* material and will produce the desired effect if followed carefully.

What is "Progressive Mobilization?"

Have you ever been in bed with the flu for a few days or a week? Have you ever climbed four flights of stairs after a considerable period of inactivity?

What did you feel like when you got out of bed? What did you feel like after climbing the stairs?

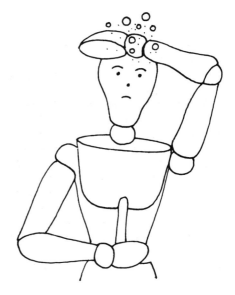

Feeling of Great Fatigue After Just a Little Exercise?

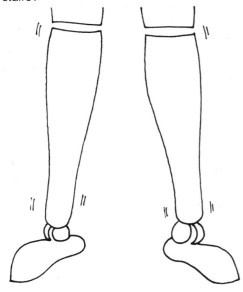

Legs Weak and Wobbly?

If you answered "yes" to these three questions, you have experienced some of the undesirable effects of bed rest or inactivity.

Note that weakness, dizziness, and fatigue *are* among the many negative effects of bed rest. Others may be contractures, pneumonia, thrombophlebitis, and pressure sores.

How can you prevent these from happening? Try using the *tools* of *Progressive Mobilization.*

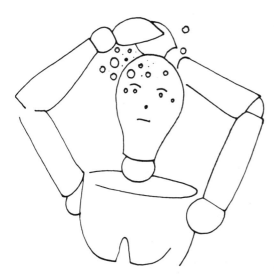

Head Dizzy?

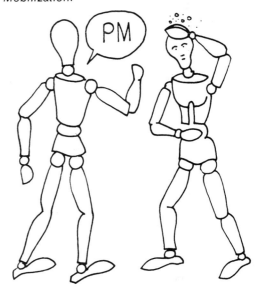

Progressive Mobilization (PM) is a program comprised of specific activities to mobilize patients and to help them gain independence. Each activity is geared to fit the individual needs and abilities of the patient. During these activities the patients are taught to move around on their own, with as little assistance from you as possible. The activities are designed to build on one another, forming a "staircase." Each step is necessary for the next step to be accomplished. For example, if the patient does not have the mobility or strength to roll over in bed alone, he will not have the mobility or strength to sit up alone. If he cannot sit up alone, he will not be able to stand up alone. At the top of this "staircase," patient independence, or a degree of independence occurs. Review the "Independent Stair-

case" shown, and note carefully each step. Each of these steps will be taught to you in detail in the remainder of this chapter.

As the steps in progressive mobilization build on one another to form a staircase, so does bed rest and/or inactivity. The difference in the two staircases is that the inactivity staircase is a *downward* one, which leads to dependence rather than independence. The *longer* the patient stays in bed or remains inactive, the less muscle strength he has, and the less he can perform activities alone. The trick to progressive mobilization is to *get the patient out of bed* and *keep him out of bed*. Review the dependent staircase below. Note each step. This staircase is the one that needs to be avoided.

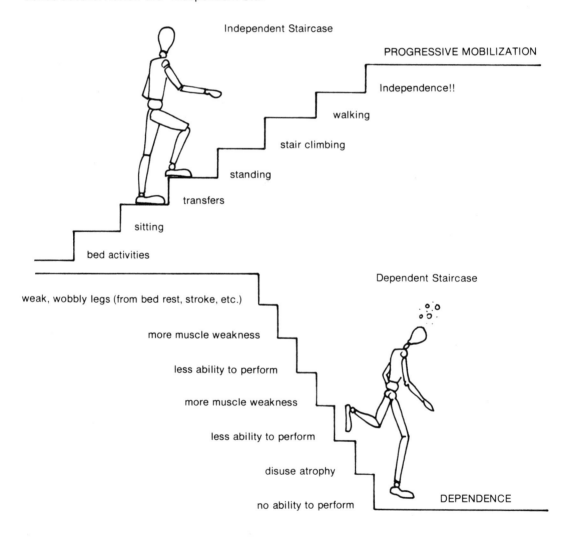

Independent Staircase

PROGRESSIVE MOBILIZATION

Independence!!

walking

stair climbing

standing

transfers

sitting

bed activities

Dependent Staircase

weak, wobbly legs (from bed rest, stroke, etc.)

more muscle weakness

less ability to perform

more muscle weakness

less ability to perform

disuse atrophy

no ability to perform

DEPENDENCE

Test for "Progressive Mobilization"

Please answer the following questions:

1. What should be the end result of progressive mobilization?

_____

2. You want the patient to have as quick a recovery to independence as possible. Name three (3) things which must be done to allow this:

a. _____

b. _____

c. _____

Answers:

1. Patient independence.

2. a. Encourage the patient to do activities without assistance as much as possible.

    b. Get him out of bed and active quickly.

    c. Keep him out of bed.

Question 2 above contains the *most important points* for the *success* of a *Progressive Mobilization Program.* If you answered correctly, go on. If not, please review before proceeding.

If people without physical disabilities experience the negative effects of bed rest or inactivity, you can certainly imagine what a patient with a disability, i.e., stroke, hip fracture, or Parkinsonism, would experience. Dr. Gerald Hirschberg in *Rehabilitation: A Manual For the Care of the Disabled and Elderly* states that the uncomplicated stroke patient can be out of bed within one to three days after the incident. In most cases, a hip fracture patient could and should be up a few days after surgery to prevent thrombophlebitis and other negative effects of bed rest.

Please remember that it is the physician's responsibility to decide the who, what, when, and where of using Progressive Mobilization. However, *you* must be aware of the benefits and value of Progressive Mobilization and *work with the physician* to help your patient toward independence as quickly as possible.

We have discovered that the dependent staircase, unfortunately, is the steeper staircase. It takes far less time for a patient to become dependent than independent or to gain back the strength lost during an excursion down the dependent staircase. The *less* you allow your patient to descend the dependent staircase, the easier and faster it will be to help him become independent again.

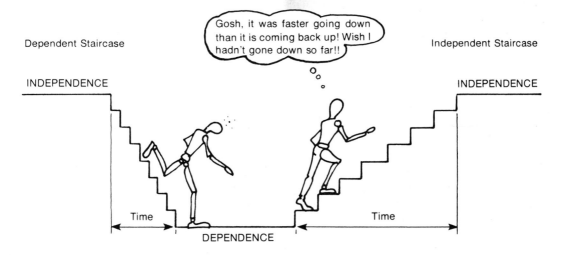

1. Who would order a program of progressive mobilization?

_____

2. Now that you know the benefits of progressive mobilization, would you remind your physician of the importance of rapid institution of progressive mobilization?

_____

If you answered (1) "The Physician" and (2) "Yes," we are pleased.

By using the methods that will be presented in the remainder of this chapter, we have found that the adverse effects encountered by inactivity or bed rest greatly outweigh the chances taken with early mobilization of the patient. Thus, Progressive Mobilization is the answer!

Before we go on—REMEMBER:

1. The undesirable effects of bed rest are progressive weakness and fatigue, which can lead to a state of dependence.
2. Progressive mobilization is a program of activities to help produce independence in your patients.
3. The quicker the program is instituted, the less loss there is of the patient's ability to perform.
4. The patient must perform the activity alone or with minimal assistance.
5. You must work *with* the physician.
6. Strength is lost faster than it can be built up.

The purpose of this chapter is to instruct you in specific techniques that will enhance your patients' independence. In the next section we shall discuss some safety factors that should play a definite part in your nursing care.

Tools to Promote Patient Safety During Treatment

Ignoring these factors might prove hazardous both for your health and the health of your patients. So, pay close attention!

We have selected three tools which should be used as guides to prevent problems during mobilization activities. They are as follows:

1. observing for cardiac symptoms,
2. monitoring the pulse, and
3. using proper body mechanics.

In applying rehabilitation concepts to general nursing care these three tools are of utmost importance. The reasons are as follows:

1. Progressive Mobilization activities often prove to be very strenuous for your patients;
2. it takes more energy for the patient to move around on his own than to be moved by you; and
3. patients often need a great deal of assistance as they start Progressive Mobilization activities.

TOOL 1: Observing for Cardiac Symptoms

Whether young or old, even a short stay in bed for disabled patients makes it difficult to perform some of the Progressive Mobilization activities without stress.

Note: *Always observe for cardiac symptoms in your patients.*

Easily Observed *Cardiac Symptoms:*

- Shortness of breath
- Substernal chest pain—left arm pain
- Skin temperature—cold sweat
- Nausea
- Skin color—pale or flushed
- Dizziness—syncope (fainting)
- Diaphoresis (sweating)

Observe your patient for these signs first *at rest* and then during each mobilization activity. If any occur, allow the patient to stop the activity and rest. The signs should reverse themselves readily. If they do, make note of them and continue the activity at a lower level, more slowly and, perhaps, with more assistance, so the activity is not as strenuous.

If any of the signs occur and do not reverse themselves readily at rest the activity should be stopped and the physician notified. He should determine if the activity should be continued or the pace of it changed.

Test for Tool 1

1. Name two (2) cardiac symptoms. a. _____
                                 b. _____
2. What should you do if cardiac symptoms occur during Progressive Mobilization activities?
   a. _____
   b. _____
   c. _____
   d. _____
3. When do you first check for cardiac symptoms?
   _____
4. Would you start a Progressive Mobilization activity if, at rest, cardiac symptoms are present?
   _____

You were correct if you answered the questions as follows:
1. If you answered any of the seven: shortness of breath, chest pain, skin temperatures, nausea, skin color, dizziness (syncope), sweating (diaphoresis).
2. Allow the patient to rest, slow down the activity, lower the level of activity, give more assistance.
3. At rest.
4. No.

TOOL 2: Monitoring the Pulse

A change in the patient's pulse rate is an important cardiac symptom. We deliberately left it out of the list of cardiac symptoms because we wanted to discuss it in terms of pulse monitoring. Pulse monitoring is the method of watching the pulse rate during Progressive Mobilization activities. It is an indication of the patient's tolerance to a particular activity. As with other cardiac symptoms, the pulse response would indicate whether the exercise should be continued, decreased, stopped temporarily, or permanently discontinued. The two important items to observe about the pulse at this time are:

1. the speed of the pulse, or pulse rate.
2. the rhythm of the pulse.

The pulse rate should be taken *first at rest*—before any activity is begun. This will be labeled as the resting pulse. After this is determined, you would begin the activity and take the pulse rate at the completion of each activity.

1. When should the pulse rate be taken?
   a. _____
   b. _____
2. What are the two (2) important items to observe regarding the pulse?

a. _____
b. _____

Answers:

1. a. At rest   b. After activity
2. a. Rhythm   b. Speed or rate

The next section, *How to Take the Pulse Rate,* is written primarily for nonprofessional people. If you are a nurse, OT, PT, or physician, you might like to review it as a teaching tool for your nonprofessional assistants. If not, turn to page 22. Important points are mentioned in these pages regarding the rhythm of the pulse.

How to Take the Pulse Rate—Take the pulse at the thumb side of the wrist on the palm or inner side of the forearm, as shown in Figure 2-1. Place your fingers at the area marked "X," and you will feel a throb there. Do not use your thumb because your thumb has its own pulse.

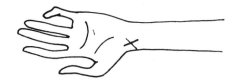

Figure 2-1

Look at the second hand on your watch and count how many beats you feel in fifteen seconds. Multiply this by four to set the pulse rate for one minute. The pulse rate is recorded per minute. If the pulse is irregular count the pulse for sixty seconds.

If the pulse rate cannot be found at the wrist, use the temple or under the jaw at the carotid artery (Figure 2-2).

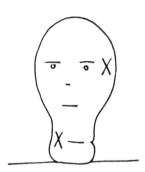

Figure 2-2

The normal resting pulse rate is 65-85 beats per minute.

Feel for your own pulse at the designated areas. Did you find it? Now figure it out for one minute. Record your pulse rate here. _____ Now find it on a friend. Everyone's pulse feels a little different. The more pulse rates you take, the easier it will be to take them.

The Rhythm of the Pulse Rate—The rhythm of the pulse should be regular. It should be an even throb—1, 2, 3, 4. An irregular pulse can be described as one which skips beats—1, _, 3, 4, or 1, _, _, 4. If a patient has an irregular pulse, the physician should be notified. This is often an indication that the activities are contraindicated, and continuation of the activity should be at his discretion.

1. *What is the normal range of the resting pulse?* _____
2. *Where should the pulse rate be taken?*
_____
_____
_____
3. *Over what period of time is the pulse rate calculated and recorded?*
_____

4. *What does an irregular pulse feel like?*
_____

Answers:

1. *65-85 beats per minute.*
2. *wrist on radial side, temple, jaw at carotid artery.*
3. *per minute.*
4. *it skips beats.*

If you answered correctly, put this knowledge to work and get to the heart of the subject.

How to Relate Pulse Taking with Activity—It is important to take the pulse rate as the patient performs the activities. It should be done in the following manner:

1. Take resting pulse.
2. Do appropriate activity.
3. Take pulse immediately following the activity.
4. Rest for two minutes. Take pulse again.
5. Repeat every two minutes until the pulse is within ten counts of the resting count.

EXAMPLE

Pulse Rate	Normal Results
Resting	60-85
Activity	90-120+
2-minute Rest	60-95

As a general rule, most patients experience an increase in pulse rate during the course of the exercise. The amount of increase and the length of time it takes to return to the resting level are the important considerations.

Complete the following exercise:

1. Take your resting pulse _____.
2. Stand up and jog in place for two minutes.
3. Take your pulse immediately after activity
_____.
4. Take your pulse after two minutes rest
_____.
5. Take your pulse after four minutes rest
_____.
6. Take your pulse after six minutes rest
_____.

Did your pulse rate change?
Did you get a good break from sitting?

Test for Tool 2

Please answer the questions below.

1. *Name five steps in taking a pulse rate in relation to activity.*
   a. _____.
   b. _____.
   c. _____.
   d. _____.
   e. _____.
2. *What two factors are the important considerations of pulse rate with activity?*
   a. _____.
   b. _____.

Answers:

1. a. *Take a resting pulse,*
   b. *Do appropriate activity,*
   c. *Take pulse immediately after activity,*
   d. *Resting for two minutes—take pulse again, and*
   e. *Repeat every two minutes until return to the rest level.*
2. a. *Amount of increase,*
   b. *Length of time to return to resting level.*

If you missed the answers review the information and try the practice cycle again. Remember you must do this pulse monitoring with *all* your patients during their activities. Once you answer correctly move on—there is more information about this important subject.

An increase of twenty beats per minute during exercise is acceptable as normal. It should ideally return to the resting rate (within ten beats per minute) within two minutes of the cessation of activity. If this does not occur after six minutes following the cessation of exercise, the physician should be notified and exercise halted until he determines if the activity should be resumed or carried out at a lower level.

The more difficult an activity is for the patient the more it will stress his heart and the higher his pulse rate will be. During a strenuous exercise such as walking, stair climbing, or stand-ups, a rise in the pulse rate of up to fifty beats, or about 122 beats per minute would be considered *satisfactory*. At a fifty-beat per minute increase or more the activity should be stopped, the patient should rest for a period of time, and later the activity should be adjusted for less exertion by the patient. This is done by doing the activity slower, by doing it for a shorter period of time, or by giving the patient greater assistance. If the pulse rate increases too much each time the activity is performed, regardless of the level at which the patient is exercising, then the particular activities are too difficult for the patient and should be stopped. A similar course of action should be taken if a patient develops an irregular pulse during the course of the exercises or activity.

It would be considered *unsatisfactory* if, during the activity of *sitting in a wheelchair*, the patient's pulse rate increased fifty beats or to about 122 per minute. Sitting in a chair is as important as any other activity on the independent staircase, but the patient *cannot be allowed the same pulse rise* as he can during strenuous exercise. *Sitting is often very stressful to the dehabilitated patient.* Frequently this patient cannot even roll over in bed alone without a tremendous rise in pulse rate, but he must get out of bed to gain any strength at all.

As a companion to exercise, a patient's sitting tolerance parallels his ability to progress up the steps of independence. Table 2-1 is a sitting tolerance schedule which, if followed carefully, produces a rapid increase in the patient's general strength.

TABLE 2-1
Sitting Tolerance Schedule

DAY	TIME OF DAY	ACTIVITY
No. 1	9:00 a.m. or 10:00 a.m.	Patient *sits* in chair or wheelchair for 15 minutes
	1:00 p.m. or 2:00 p.m.	Same activity for 30 minutes
	5:00 p.m. or 6:00 p.m.	Same activity for 45 minutes
No. 2	9:00 a.m. or 10:00 a.m.	Patient sits in chair or wheelchair for 1 hour
	1:00 p.m. or 2:00 p.m.	Same activity for 1 hour 15 minutes
	5:00 p.m. or 6:00 p.m.	Same activity for 1 hour 30 minutes
No. 3	9:00 a.m. or 10:00 a.m.	Same activity for 2 hours
	1:00 p.m. or 2:00 p.m.	Same activity for 2 hours 15 minutes
	5:00 p.m. or 6:00 p.m.	Same activity for 2 hours 30 minutes
No. 4	9:00 a.m. or 10:00 a.m.	Same activity for 3 hours
	1:00 p.m. or 2:00 p.m.	Same activity for 3 hours 15 minutes
	5:00 p.m. or 6:00 p.m.	Same activity for 3 hours 30 minutes

Continue the schedule progressively as shown in Table 2-1 until the patient is out of bed as follows:

- out of bed 5 hours in morning,
- nap 1 to 1-1/2 hours after lunch, and
- out of bed 5 hours in the afternoon.

The ultimate *goal* is for the patient to be *out of bed from twelve to fourteen hours per day.*

All patients will not start at the same point on the sitting tolerance schedule. To determine where to start, a number of things must be considered:

1. How much time the patient has been up previously. (If the patient cannot tell you this information, the family or chart notes should.)
2. If this cannot be determined, start the patient according to Day 1 on the schedule.
3. The pulse response of the patient and other cardiac symptoms.

The most important determination of the sitting tolerance of the patient is his pulse response. Patients will beg to go back to bed; but as long as their pulse is satisfactory with-

out the other cardiac symptoms, they *must stay up.* We tell them, "You might feel tired, but your heart is not tired yet. So you can sit up longer." Often in early rehabilitation of a patient, only bed exercises and sitting can be tolerated. If the dehabilitated patient experiences syncope when first sitting on the edge of the bed (prior to the transfer to a chair), the blood pressure should be taken. If hypotensive, support stockings should be considered. If the patient still experiences syncope while sitting upright, neurochairs or a recliner wheelchair might have to be utilized. As the patient tolerates a ninety-degree angle in the neurochair without dizziness, he can be mobilized to a regular wheelchair. (See Chapter 6 for neurochair and recliner wheelchair information.)

A patient's out of bed tolerance has to increase to a certain amount before he can go any further on his strengthening program. As mentioned previously, a patient's sitting tolerance and ability to strengthen correspond very closely. The patient who still continually begs to go to bed might be able to walk only a few feet, while the patient who sits up all day is able to walk around the block.

Sitting time and the sitting pulse response are evaluated in the following manner:

1. If the pulse is 100 beats per minute or below without any other cardiac symptoms, the patient should stay up. Remember that with transferring the patient into the chair or even with lifting him, his pulse rate may increase above this level. But if within six minutes after the transfer activity his pulse is at his resting rate, or 100 or below, continued sitting as planned is fine.
2. If the pulse remains higher than 100 beats per minute (or 104-108 per minute or above), the patient should be returned to bed. The activity should be tried again later at the next scheduled time.

To summarize:

1. Take pulse rates often.
2. Do activities for short periods of time.
3. Let your patient rest between activities— five minutes will usually be sufficient.
4. A strenuous activity after rest will not cause as much stress on the patient as it would if done immediately following another activity.
5. Do not let the patient return to bed too quickly.
6. If the pulse rate sitting is 100 or below, the patient should stay out of bed.
7. If the pulse rate sitting is over 100, try sitting the patient later.
8. Keep patients up longer each time they are out of bed.

Test for Tool 2

Please answer the following five questions:

1. *What should be done if the patient develops an irregular pulse or a pulse increase greater than fifty beats/minute? Name three steps.*

   _____
   _____
   _____
   _____

2. *What is the longest length of time a pulse rate could remain high (above resting level) and still be okay?* _____

3. *How do you adjust an activity to a lower output level without stopping the activity? Name two ways.*

   a. _____
   b. _____
   _____

4. *How long should the patient be able to sit up at one session by the end of Day No. 3?*
   _____

5. *What does the comment mean: "Your heart's not tired yet so you can stay up longer."*
   _____
   _____
   _____
   _____
   _____

Answers:

1. *Stop activity, rest for a period of time, adjust the activity.*
2. *Six minutes.*
3. *Make activity periods shorter, help the patient more, do activity slower.*
4. *2 hours, 30 minutes.*
5. *That a patient's pulse is 100 or below, strong, steady and there are no other cardiac symptoms.*

Western Iowa Tech-IMC

11786

TOOL 3: *Using Proper Body Mechanics*

An important aspect of safety in the application of Progressive Mobilization is the knowledge and proper use of body mechanics both for you and for your patients. In addition to using correct body mechanics for safety, you will be teaching your patients to use their bodies in such a way that the mechanics of the body assist and make the activities easier for them.

In most activities related to patient care the four *basic principles of body mechanics* are:

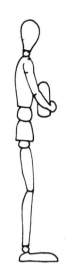

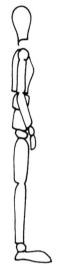

1. Keep your back straight.

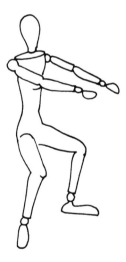

2. Bend your knees, squat, and use your thigh muscles.

3. Hold the object as close to you as possible.

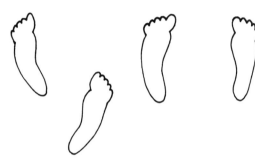

4. Keep a wide base of support by placing one foot in front of the other or sideways.

To avoid situations that are dangerous to you and your patient, follow these four principles and "look at yourself" while working.

The following dialogue might serve as a good example of what *NOT* to do.

NURSE: Mr. Smith, can I help you get out of bed?

MR. SMITH: Oh, yes!

Mr. Smith reaches up with both arms ...

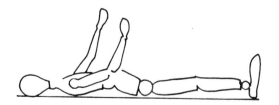

The nurse bends over. Mr. Smith puts his arms around the neck of the nurse whose hands are placed under his shoulders.

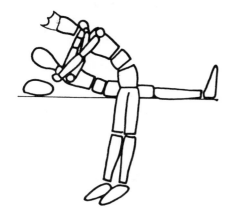

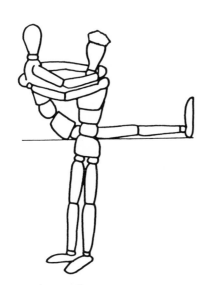

The nurse then pulls up.

Review the four principles of body mechanics and *look at the nurse!*

What is wrong? (Circle the appropriate answer for each item).

1. The nurse *has* or *has not* kept the back straight.
2. The nurse *has* or *has not* held the object close.

3. The nurse *has* or *has not* bent the knees.
4. The nurse *has* or *has not* spread the feet to keep a wide base of support.

Answers: None of the principles of proper body mechanics has been followed. Review this drawing:

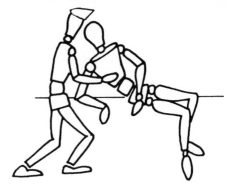

This is the proper procedure for getting a patient out of bed.

Two Activities to Try

1. Put a book on the floor.
   a. Stand up, put your feet close together until they touch each other, bend your knees, keep your back straight, and pick up the book. Stand up.
   b. Now get a wide base of support by spreading your feet forward or sideways. Bend your knees, keep your back straight, and pick up the book. Stand up.

You felt off balance using method (a), didn't you? Your feet did not give you a good stable foundation in that position. Method (b) is the more stable position. (If the book had been a person who moved suddenly, over you'd go!)
   Now try this:

2. Place a book on the table.
   a. Bend your elbows and pick up the book (Figure 2-3).
   b. Now keep your elbows straight and pick up the book. The book felt heavier with your elbows straight, didn't it? This is explained by the physics principle that a weight is heavier at the end of a long lever arm.

Keeping your arms straight created a long lever arm.

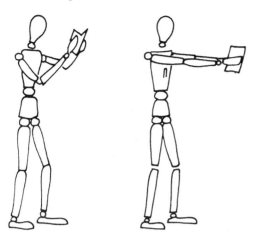

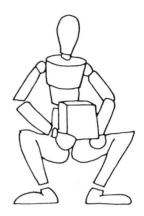

Figure 2-6

Note: Short Lever Arm
Correct Method of Lifting

Figure 2-3   **Figure 2-4**

c. When you lift a patient be sure to bend your elbows and hold him close so that he will be lighter. When you bend over at the hips, and reach down to the floor to pick an object up, you are again creating a long lever arm (Figure 2-5). See the following pictures of the correct and incorrect method of lifting an object off the floor. (Figures 2-5 and 2-6.)

Test for Tool 3

Considering the principles of body mechanics:

1. *Circle the correct picture of how to get Mr. Smith from a seated position to a standing position.*
2. *Under each picture, list the correct or incorrect procedures the nurse is using.*

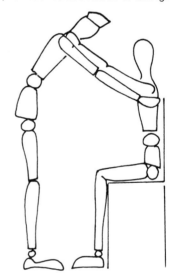

A.

_____

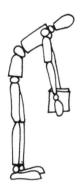

Figure 2-5

Note: Long Lever Arm
Incorrect Method of Lifting

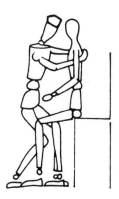

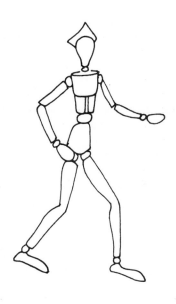

B.

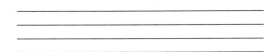

Nurse "B" *did* remember . . .

Answers:

1. *You should have circled "B".*
2. A. *Back is bent, legs are straight, no wide base of support, object not close.*
   B. *Object close, knees bent, back straight, wide base of support.*

Remember to keep these principles in mind whenever working with a patient, making a bed, or lifting something off the floor at work or at home. They will prevent back injuries!

Other safety points will be mentioned as the activities are presented. There are two precautions which apply to *all* situations:

1. If you are not sure that you can carry out an activity alone because of the weight or the condition of the patient, discontinue activity and get help.

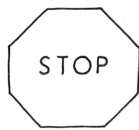

2. *Always* work in an area where you can *summon* help if you need it.

Continue reading to determine how to coordinate all of this information.

Where to Begin Progressive Mobilization?

Have you ever seen two patients alike?

On May 25th, three stroke patients arrived at your hospital. Mr. A. is unconscious. He is unable to move at all. He is medically stable.

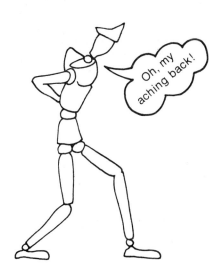

Nurse "A" *did not* remember . . .

Mr. B. is awake, alert, talkative, and wants to get up immediately. He is accustomed to being up all day. He can move his right arm and leg easily although the right side is not quite as strong as the left. Mr. C. is awake, but confused, disoriented, completely paralyzed on his right side, and weak on the left side. His family tells us that he has sat up in a wheelchair for thirty minutes twice a day.

Now, what do you do?

You know what Progressive Mobilization is, but how do you apply this idea? Remember the Independence Staircase? Remember the Sitting Tolerance Schedule? Keep them in your mind and use them as a guide to evaluate your patient. Use them as a check-out list when you see a patient for the first time. Check the patient out on every step of the Independence Staircase. If he passes Step 1, good; go on to Step 2, 3. If he falters on Step 4 . . . that is where the work begins . . . . As you study the steps in detail you will be able to tell quickly what your patient can do and where you need to go from there.

By testing the patient in each activity you can determine

1. whether the patient can do the activity, or
2. if he needs to be taught to do the activity, or
3. if he needs to practice several activities simultaneously.

Here are some questions regarding where to begin Progressive Mobilization activities. In answering these questions you may refer back to the drawing of the Independence Staircase (p. 18), to the Sitting Tolerance Schedule (p. 24) and to the descriptions of Misters A., B., and C. Please name the step in the Progressive Mobilization program at which you would start each patient.

1. You asked Mr. A. to move in bed alone. He could not respond to your command. _____

2. You asked Mr. B. to move in bed. He did it easily. You asked him to sit up. He jumped up out of bed the minute the siderails went down. He stood up easily but after a few steps his right knee gave way. _____
_____

3. You asked Mr. C. to move in bed. He did. You asked him to sit up. He needed moderate assistance getting to a sitting position and after he sat a few seconds he started leaning badly to the left. _____
_____

Do you think you put your patient on the correct step?

1. *Bed Activities.* Even at this point it looks as if you are going to have to do all the bed activities for him until he starts gaining consciousness and can start helping himself. He should sit in a neurochair for fifteen minutes.
2. *Walking step.* You could return to the standing step. Even though he did it easily you could use the exercise to strengthen the patient's right knee. This will be clearer after you read the discussion of the activities. The patient should sit up all day.
3. *Sitting.* Start on Day 2—sit up in wheelchair for forty-five minutes and continue as scheduled. Practice sitting balance. He does not have enough trunk control or general strength to proceed to standing yet.

How did you do?

If you will reread this section after you have learned how to do all of the activities, the decision of where to start Progressive Mobilization will be even clearer.

Now, complete the following Posttest for this unit.

Posttest for What is "Progressive Mobilization?"

Write your answers in the space provided.

1. *What is a Progressive Mobilization Program?* _____
2. *At what rate should a patient's time sitting in a chair be increased?* _____

3. Your patient has casts on both wrists. Where can you feel his pulse?
_____

4. Mr. Jones has been in bed for one day. Mrs. Smith has been in bed for three weeks. If their diagnoses are the same, which patient would be rehabilitated the quickest?_____
Why?_____

5. In a Progressive Mobilization program, when should you first take the patient's pulse rate?

6. Mr. Jones has a pulse rate of 132 when resting in bed. You are supposed to start Progressive Mobilization activities. What should you do? (The chart said his pulse rate averages 85.)
a. _____ b. _____

7. You have been exercising Mr. Jones. His resting pulse rate was 80.
a. After the activity it is 100. What would you do?
(1) _____ (2) _____
b. After the activity it is 130. What would you do?
(1) _____ (2) _____

8. Mr. Jones is weak, very heavy and he needs to get to the bathroom. What would you do?
_____

9. The Independence Staircase can be used as an _____

10. State the relationship between the steps of the Independence Staircase.
_____

11. If a patient's pulse is 99 and he complains of being tired while sitting in a chair but has no other cardiac symptoms, what would you do? _____

12. You are going to lift a two-year-old child off the floor. Applying good body mechanics, how are you going to hold him? _____

Answers:

1. Activities to gain independence and mobility.
2. Each time should be fifteen minutes longer.
3. Feel it at the temple or at the jaw at the carotid artery.
4. Mr. Jones. Because he has had less time to become weak from staying in bed.
5. At rest.
6. a. Don't do the activity.   b. Notify the doctor.
7. a. (1) Let him rest.   (2) Continue the exercise.
   b. (1) Let him rest.   (2) Stop the activity.
8. Get someone to help you with him.
9. Evaluation guide.
10. Each step is necessary for the next to be accomplished.
11. Reassure him that he is all right and keep him sitting up.
12. Hold him close to your body.

If you answered eleven or twelve correctly, excellent—go on.

If you answered eight or nine correctly—that is satisfactory, but please review.

If you answered less than seven correctly, please repeat this unit.

You are now prepared to learn more about specific Progressive Mobilization activities. The objective of the instruction in this chapter is the following: Given details of patient history and clinical diagnosis, you should be able to promote the patient's mobility by using the proper activities and assistive devices. Specifically, once you have completed this chapter you should be able to:

1. identify the steps in each of the activities,
2. perform the activities yourself,
3. demonstrate the activities to the patient,
4. select activities appropriate to the particular patient,

5. *select assistive devices* appropriate to the particular patient, and
6. teach the patient the activity.

(The student should be able to perform a certain activity or group of activities *for the clinical instructor*, or, if a clinical instructor is not present, your patient should *demonstrate the activity to you* as you stand by. If the patient is able or knows how to perform the activity after you have taught him, you have fulfilled this objective).

Each step of the Independence Staircase represents a specific activity. Each of the following activities will be discussed and carefully explained to you:

a. bed activities,
b. sitting,
c. transfers,
d. standing,
e. stair climbing, and
f. walking.

To make the descriptions of the activities more realistic and easier to follow, most of the activities are presented in the form of a dialogue using "the nurse" to represent you, and "Mr. Jones" to represent the patient. Mr. Jones and the nurse "climb" the steps on the Independence Staircase. The nurse "sets the scene," and the activities are presented. The best way to approach the study of these activities is to hold book in hand and act out each step yourself as if you were Mr. Jones.

The activities are presented in basic form. Their adatation by you in practice depends upon the diagnosis of the patient. For example, a stroke patient and a nonweight-bearing hip fracture patient would transfer using the same basic technique, except that the fractured hip patient would keep the involved foot off the floor.

Table 2-2 lists some common diagnoses with their accompanying major functional limitations. These limitations are the ones that are important to consider carefully when adapting a particular exercise to a particular patient and when selecting activities for your patient. (See Chapter 1 or reference materials for more detailed explanation of these disabilities.) Table 2-2 contains only a *few considerations,* but these *pertain most directly* to the topic of Progressive Mobilization Activities.

Take a break—then join Mr. Jones and his nurse in "bed activities" for their climb *Up the Independence Staircase.*

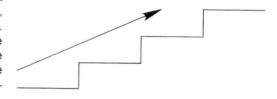

TABLE 2-2

Common Diagnoses and Accompanying Disabilities

Type of Disability	Major Functional Limitations
1. Stroke	Paralyzed upper and lower extremities on one side. Partially paralyzed upper and lower extremity on one side. Hemianopsia—the ability to see only out of one side of each eye. Poor balance.
2. Fractured hip: surgically pinned.	Unable to put weight on involved leg.
3. Fractured hip — closed reduction.	Same as above.
4. Austin-Moore prosthesis or total hip prosthesis.	Able to bear weight as specified by physician.
5. Arthritis	May have limited motion in joints. May have painful joints.
6. Parkinsonism	Rigidity. Limited range of motion.

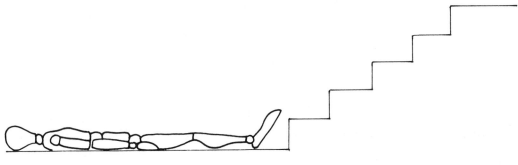

Bed Positioning

Bed Activities

The first step on the Independence Staircase is bed activity. These activities should be started as soon as the patient is hospitalized. Because they are actually a part of every day nursing care, these activities are readily initiated. Before we list them visualize this:

You have been assigned to give Mr. Jones a bath. When you enter the room, you notice that Mr. Jones has slid down too low in the bed. What should you do? You have two choices after lowering the head of the bed:

1. Pull him up in bed yourself or call a nurse to help. Both of you then pull Mr. Jones up in bed. Mr. Jones does NONE of the work. Or,
2. Tell Mr. Jones where to hold onto the bed and how to push with his feet. Then you and Mr. Jones work together to move him up in bed.

See the picture? One task, two different approaches. If you use Approach No. 2, the next day Mr. Jones will be able to help you again, and help more because he will be stronger from having done the activity on the first day. Soon, Mr. Jones might be able to move up in bed alone.

Remember the theory of Progressive Mobilization as stated in our introduction? The sooner the patient is encouraged and taught to move around on his own, the sooner his recovery comes about, and the sooner he is independent again.

There are five activities that can be listed as bed activities. They are as follows:

1. Bed positioning.
2. Range of motion (ROM).
   a. Passive range of motion.
   b. Active range of motion.
   c. Functional range of motion.
3. Moving up and down in bed.
4. Moving sideways.
5. Rolling over in bed.

Bed positioning and *passive* range of motion activities are preventative. They are important in preventing joint and muscle contractures. They are not done actively by the patient and, therefore, will not make him stronger. If the patient is out of bed and moving about, the need for these two activities diminishes greatly. Remember:

1. Only by doing activities himself does the patient gain strength.
2. Use the Sitting Tolerance Schedule (Table 2-1) as soon as possible and *while* the patient is learning the different steps to independence.

Bed Positioning

(Refer also to the chapter on Pressure Sores.)

Bed positioning is important if the patient cannot get out of bed yet or is in bed for long periods of time. When positioning the patient, you should think of him as a person who will be walking some day. Consequently, his arms, legs, and head should be positioned in such a way that deformities do not result from the way he lies in bed. This is why positioning is so important for a bed-bound patient. Let us now discuss the different parts of the body and how they should or should not be positioned.

Area to be Positioned: The Head

Correct Position

Use one flat pillow.

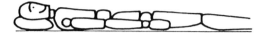

Incorrect Position

Do not use a stack of pillows.

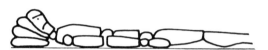

Why

The head could get stiff in a forward, flexed position and the patient's posture would be out of alignment. He would be looking down at the floor all of the time. Do not give in to patients who beg to be propped up. Frequently patients beg to be propped up. This is because with age and some medical conditions, the head naturally assumes a forward flexed position. Some of this cannot be avoided. Do not initiate the habit of propping the patient up in bed. If a patient is comfortable lying flat, leave him flat and encourage him to stay that way.

Area to be Positioned: The Knees

Correct Position

Keep the knees straight.

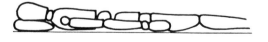

Incorrect Position

Do not put pillows under the knees that hold them flexed.

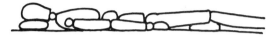

Why

Pillows under the knees produce flexion of the knee and also flexion of the hip joints. This position held for continued periods of time will produce shortening of the hamstrings and hip flexors and stiffening of the respective joints. When the patient tries to walk he will not be able to straighten up and will probably look like this . . .

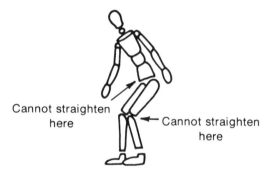

Cannot straighten here

Cannot straighten here

If his head is bent down also, he looks like this:

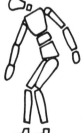

Could you walk this way? Do you recognize any patients you have seen? Parkinsonism and arthritic patients are the most hindered by these two problems.

Area to be Positioned: The Legs

Correct Position

Keep the toes and knees pointed toward the ceiling. Place a rolled bath mat under hips at a diagonal as shown to keep the proper position.

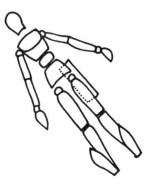

Incorrect Position

Do not let the leg remain in an externally rotated (or leg rolled outward) position. Do not place sandbags along the leg to hold the leg in the correct position.

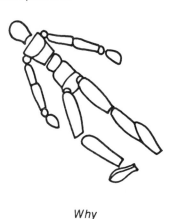

Why

Outward rotation of the leg in a supine or backlying position is a natural occurrence for a patient in bed, and one need not be concerned for most patients. But for the stroke patient or a patient with a fractured hip this is an important consideration. If the leg is not kept in the position described here, the hip will tighten in an outward position. When the patient starts walking, he will look like this . . .

toes and knees cannot point straight ahead.

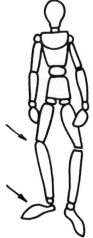

This makes gait very difficult or impossible. External rotation of the leg is a motion of the hip joint and correction of it is most effective when made at the hip.

Area to be Positioned: The Ankles

Correct Position

Keep ankle flexible at least to a 90° angle.

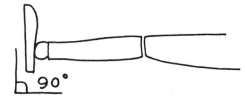

Incorrect Position

Do not let heel cord (gastrocnemius muscle) shorten.

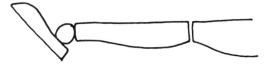

Why

If a patient cannot dorsiflex his feet to at least a 90° angle he will walk on his toes all the time—this is very debilitating. Stroke, Parkinsonism, and arthritic patients seem to have the most difficulty with this. Instruct the patient to move his ankle up and down by himself many times during the day. *Active movement of the ankle will keep the heel cord from tightening and strengthen the ankle muscles.* The nurse does passive ROM on the ankle each time she is in the room. *This prevents tightening of the ankle and corresponding muscles.* Keep covers loose over feet. Do not tighten sheets down on feet. *Tight sheets pull the feet down into plantar flexion. Also prevents the patient from moving his feet by himself. Footboards are effective if patients do not move away from them.*

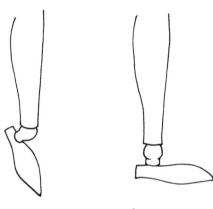

tight heel cord   normal

Area to be Positioned: Arms and Hands

Correct Position

Keep arms abducted from the body.

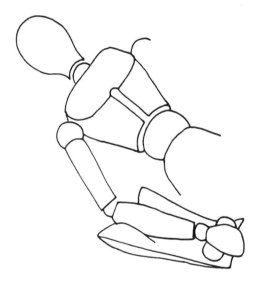

Incorrect Position

Do not keep arms tightly pressed against sides.

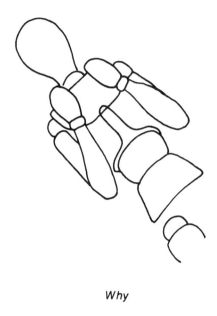

Why

To prevent pressure sores. Do not allow the elbows to be kept maximally flexed. *To prevent contractures of elbow muscles.* Move arms often into different positions. *During the course of the day, the shoulder can be positioned at different points of ROM of the joint. (Positions will be discussed more in ROM exercise section).* Elevate arms and hands. *To reduce or prevent further swelling in hands and arms.* Place hands stretched out flat against bed or pillow keeping wrist in a neutral position or place a roll in the hand. *To keep the wrist and fingers flexible and in a functional position. If shoulders, elbows, wrists and fingers have contractures, functional use of them is impaired. If limitations occur in the upper extremities, the patient may not be able to feed or dress himself and may not be able to use walking aids (i.e., crutches or walkers), if they are needed.*

To reinforce the need for proper positioning, I would like to tell you about a patient I saw years ago. She was an obese woman who had diabetes and bilateral strokes. She was alert and in obvious discomfort. She lay in the fetal position. Her arms were tightly adducted against her body and her fingers were bent into tight fists. Her knees and hips were flexed and tightly adducted. She had developed pressure sores everywhere that the surfaces of her body touched each other. We could not move her arms away from her body and she had sores under her armpits and under her breasts where her hands pressed hard against her.

The need for getting this woman moved around was very evident to me. But, when we started to treat her, we found that nothing could be done to help her. A great deal could have been accomplished if Progressive Mobilization had occurred when she first became ill. Need I say more?

Bed positioning is a difficult job. It is much easier to work with a patient who is out of bed, so your goal should be to get him up and around. I hope that from this discussion you can see the *need to position* your newly hospitalized and bed-bound patient. If you do not, you could be responsible for deformities that could possibly prevent his independence.

Test for Bed Positioning

1. *Which two joints can stiffen if you place pillows under a patient's knees when he is in bed?*
   a. _____ b. _____
2. *Where do you put the roll to prevent outward movement of the whole leg?*
   _____
3. *What are the two best ways to prevent a tight heel cord or ankle stiffness for a bed-bound patient?*
   a. _____
   b. _____

If you answered:

1. *a. the hip, b. the knee,*
2. *at the hip (remember external rotation is a hip motion),*
3. *have the patient do the motion himself and passive range of motion,*

you were correct.

We have discussed bed positioning from a back lying position and now that you know the theory of what position is best for each joint, you should apply it appropriately when your patient is in a different position.

The trick to positioning is *good alignment of the body* in all positions. Changing positions often (at least every two hours) helps prevent contractures and pressure sores. (Remember also to review Chapter 9).

The Theory of Range of Motion— Passive, Active, and Functional

Range of motion (ROM) is a concept that refers to the amount of movement present in a joint. This motion is present in relation to the different planes of the body. Basically, there are nine types of motion for joints:

1. flexion (bending),
2. extension (straightening),
3. abduction (motion away from the midline of the body),
4. adduction (motion toward the midline of the body),
5. circumduction (circular motion),
6. supination,
7. pronation,
8. plantar flexion (downward motion of the foot at the ankle joint), and
9. dorsiflexion (upward motion of foot at the ankle joint)

Some joints can exhibit more of these movements than other joints.

There are three ways of performing range of motion activities. They are as follows:

1. *Passive ROM*. In this activity the *nurse moves* the extremity in such a way that full motion occurs at the joint. For example: moving the arm produces ROM at the shoulder.

2. *Active ROM*. In this activity all movements are the same as passive ROM except that the *patient uses his muscles* to do the moving.

3. *Functional Activities for ROM*. The patient rolls over in bed, moves up in bed, sits up, stands, gets dressed, etc. When he pulls himself up in bed, he reaches over his head to the top of the bed which produces flexion of the shoulder. Many functional activities produce full ROM of the joints.

Here is a breakdown of what each type of ROM will accomplish:

PASSIVE ROM	ACTIVE ROM	FUNCTIONAL ACTIVITIES FOR ROM
Keeps joints limber	Keeps joints limber	Keeps joints limber
Keeps muscles limber	Keeps muscle limber	Keeps muscles limber
		Strengthens
	Strengthens	*Accomplishes a necessary activity*

Notice that only passive ROM does *not* strengthen. The proper use of ROM activities is very important. It is a physiological fact that muscles will become stronger only if they do work. Passive ROM makes the nurse stronger—not the patient.

Can you see why our goal is to have the patient move around by himself? When a patient is active, the need for most specific ROM activities is greatly diminished or eliminated. The importance of ROM, how it relates to strengthening and functional activities, and how to do it will now be discussed.

The Importance of Range of Motion

We discussed in the bed positioning section good positioning to prevent contractures. Stressed in that section was the fact that, if contractures were allowed to develop, functional abilities would be greatly impaired. Movement of the joints and muscles also prevents contractures. ROM is a method, like positioning, to guarantee an absence of contractures and to promote rehabilitation. For example, if a patient's elbow becomes contracted he may not be able to dress himself. If knee contractures develop he may not be able to walk.

How to Use Range of Motion Activities—
1. *Use range of motion as an evaluative guide.* First do passive range of motion on your patient to find areas that seem tight. Once these areas are located, use the ROM techniques to loosen them and to keep them loose. Then, again by using ROM activities, test the patient's strength. Remember, never do range of motion "passively" when the patient can "actively" do it himself. Assist him to do the range of motion fully (active-assistive range of motion). This will eventually make the patient strong enough to do ROM activities alone (active ROM). When he has *some* active strength he may be able to use range of motion in his daily activities, e.g., rolling over in bed. When strengthening by using functional activities, be sure to give the patient *time to try* to perform the activity or to utilize his muscle strength maximally. Also proper instructions in utilizing functional activities are very important. (You will learn that later.)

2. *Do not overemphasize range of motion.* ROM can be done, effectively, one time per day, in conjunction with the following nursing activities:

a. *Bed bath.* Instead of moving the arm just enough to squeeze in a wash cloth, move the arm out to the side and back over the patient's head as far as it will go. This will accomplish two things at once—range of motion and a good bath. Also, have the patient roll over by himself. This will help to strengthen his muscles and keep his joints limber.

b. *Bed positioning* (as already discussed).

c. *Mobilization.* When a patient sits, his hips and knees are bent. When he lies down his hips and knees are straight. (See Figures 2-7 and 2-8.) He gets range of motion on his hips and knees in a chair.

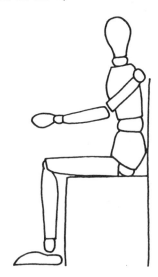

Figure 2-7

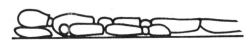

Figure 2-8

When the patient sits with his feet flat on the floor or on the foot plate of a wheelchair he is getting ROM to his ankles (heel cords are being stretched). NOTE: Standing and walking are the very best ROM exercises for heel cords. Do you see that, if you take note of these activities during the day, there are many daily activities that will accomplish the range of motion activities for you?

3. *Do Specific Stretching ROM on Two-Joint Muscles.* Limitation of range of motion is usually present where a muscle is tight. The muscles most likely to tighten are those that bridge (cross) two or more joints.

For example:

The Gastrocnemius:

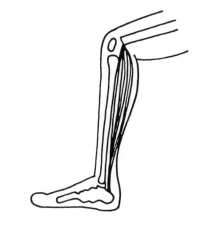

The Hamstrings:

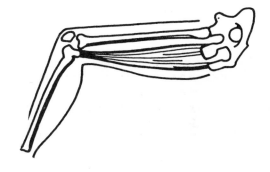

The Finger Flexors:

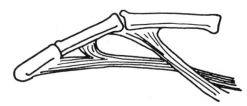

Because of this, specific stretching range of motion orders are often written for these areas. *In most other areas general functioning in daily activities will fulfill range of motion needs.*

Test for The Theory of Range of Motion

Before continuing to show you how to perform ROM activities, answer these questions to see if you understand the theory of range of motion.

1. *If your patient is bed-bound and cannot move alone at all, what type of range of motion would you do?* _____

2. *At what time during the day would you do range of motion with your patient?* _____
_____

3. *ROM activities prevent* _____
of muscles and joints.

4. *Is there a need for ROM activities when the patient is up and out of bed?*
_____

5. *Your patient has some active strength. Would he be able to roll over in bed?* _____
*Why?*_____

6. *Which muscles tend to be the tightest?*
_____

Answers:

1. *Passive ROM.*
2. *While bathing or other routine nursing activities.*
3. *Tightness, contractures.*
4. *No, not as much, perhaps only in specific areas.*
5. *Maybe; he does not need full active strength—he might be able to do some of the activity.*
6. *Muscles which bridge two joints.*

Did you answer these correctly? Review if you missed any.

Before showing you the specific directions, here are some general notes about performing ROM on a patient.

1. The patient's arms and legs should be moved gently during ROM, always within the patient's pain tolerance and the flexibility of the muscle and joints. Slow, careful movements will allow the muscles to relax in their new position and then allow further motion. There are some diagnoses where there is no pain and overzealous ROM could injure the patient, e.g. myositis ossificans.

2. Support the area to be treated. *Support the extremity above and below the joint* being moved to ensure true motion of the joint.

3. When passive ROM is given, the patient should be in the supine position to make it most effective. Self ROM activities can be performed sitting or supine. Shoulder flexion is always best supine if done passively, but it is effective in the sitting position also. Our pictures here show sit-

ting self-ROM.

4. Do each exercise five to ten times *once daily*—do ROM on problem areas more frequently (three to four times).

5. Check the motion of the involved side against the normal side to evaluate full ROM of the joints.

6. If a patient is totally bedbound, do ROM activities on all extremities.

7. When the patient can do these motions alone, the motions are called active ROM.

8. Using the motions exactly as outlined and adding a weight or resistance to the movements, one then starts progressive resistive exercise (PRE) to individual muscles. PRE, especially when the muscle is strong enough to work against gravity, enhances the strengthening of the muscle.

Functional activities serve a triple purpose: to accomplish ROM, to build strength, and to accomplish a necessary activity all at the same time. It is wonderful for a patient to be able to lift a ten-pound weight with his leg muscles, but if he cannot get out of a chair alone he is *stuck*. (Strengthening leg muscles using functional activities will be discussed later.)

Please continue now to learn how to do ROM. All these instructions can be very useful for giving home instructions for patients. They are also a ready reference for using ROM on patients later. They need not be learned in full detail now, *but do perform each movement actively yourself while reading the material.* This will help you later to evaluate ROM in the functional activities discussed.

Performing Range of Motion

The following pages show pictures and give instructions regarding passive range of motion activities. Two types of passive ROM will be compared. First you will see the nurse giving ROM to the patient who cannot do it by himself, and then you will see a hemiplegic patient giving himself daily routine ROM to his upper extremity.

Upper Extremities

ROM by Nurse

Shoulder Flexion

Starting Position: Keep arm straight
Hold arm as shown across the wrist and at the elbow: (1).

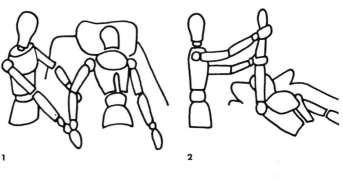

1   2

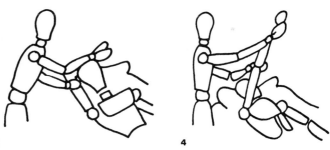

3   4

ROM Movement: Lift the arm straight over the patient's head until the arm rests flat on the bed above the head: (2)(3).

Reverse the motion and repeat: (4).

Note picture (3). Bend the patient's elbow if there is not enough room on the bed for the motion.

Hemiplegic Self-ROM

Shoulder Flexion

Starting Position: Keep arm straight
Hold wrist of affected arm with unaffected hand: (1).

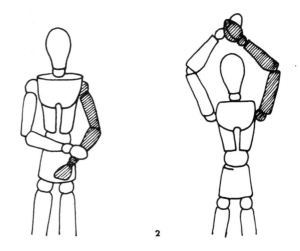

ROM Movement: Raise the arm above the head: (2).
Sit in a straight-backed chair so the patient does not tip his body.

ROM By Nurse

Shoulder Abduction

Starting Position: Keep the arms straight by the side, palm of patient's hand facing his body. Hold the arm as shown across the wrist and at the patient's elbow: (1).

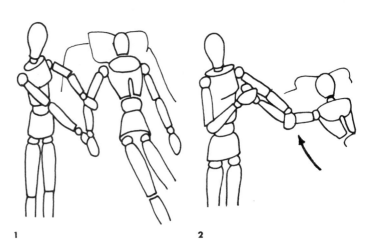

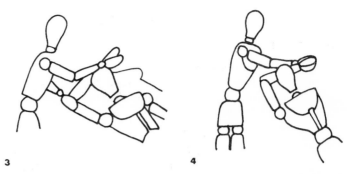

3   **4**

ROM: Keeping the arm flat on bed slide the arm sideways away from the body: (2). Keep moving the arm on the bed until the elbow touches the ear. Allow the arm to roll or turn over at about a 90° angle with the shoulder. Also bend the elbow as the arm comes up to the head if there is not enough room on the bed for the motion: (3)(4).

Hemiplegic Self-ROM

Shoulder Abduction

Starting Position: Assume cradle position by grasping the affected arm at the elbow and raise the arms to shoulder height: (1) and (2).

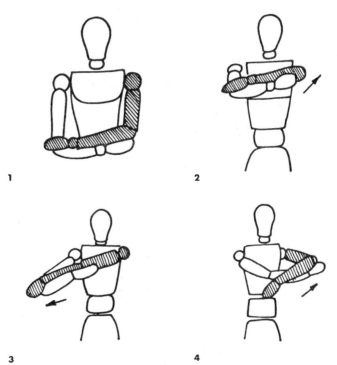

1   **2**

3   **4**

ROM: Holding the arm at shoulder height, move the arm from side to side: (3) and (4). Move only the arm—do not move the body.

ROM By Nurse

External-Internal Rotation

Starting Position: Bring the arm out from the side forming a 90° angle with the body. Keep the elbow bent to a 90° angle. Keep the upper arm on the bed. Press down on the shoulder toward the bed: (1).

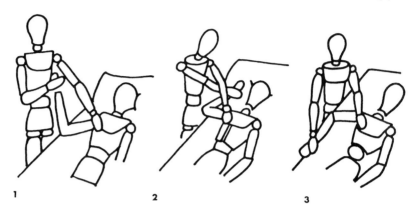

1   2   3

ROM: Move the hand gently back until the back of the hand touches the bed: (2) (external rotation). Then move the hand forward until the palm of the hand touches the bed: (3) (internal rotation).

Note: Be sure that the arm and shoulder remain in position.

Hemiplegic Self-ROM

External-Internal Rotation

Starting Position: Interlock the fingers: (1).

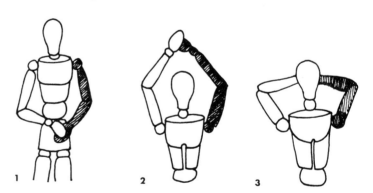

1   2   3

ROM: Lift the hand behind the neck (external rotation). Bring elbows forward, touch elbows together, and then move elbows backward (external rotation and abduction). Repeat from beginning. Also—in wheelchair:

Starting position: Position elbow of affected arm inside of wheelchair arm rest. With other hand grasp forearm of the affected extremity.

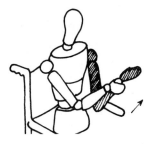

ROM: Push forearm away from body being careful that arm remains stabilized against wheelchair arm rest.

ROM By Nurse

Elbow Flexion and Extension

Starting Position: Lay patient's arm down on the bed.
Place your hands one above elbow, one at wrist.

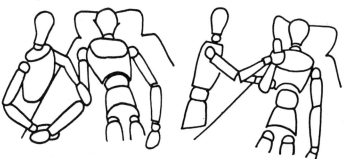

ROM: Bend arm to touch hand to shoulder. Then straighten arm completely.

Hemiplegic Self-ROM

Starting Position: Grasp affected extremity at the wrist.

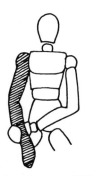

ROM: Same directions as ROM by the nurse.

ROM By Nurse

Supination and Pronation

Starting Position: Rest upper arm on bed, bend elbow to a 90° angle. Hold upper arm against the bed, hold the patient's hand at the wrist: (1).

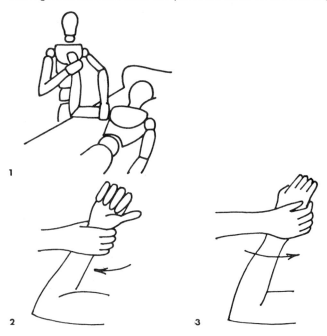

ROM: Turn the palm of the patient's hand toward his feet (pronated position) (2), then toward his face (supinated position) (3).

Hemiplegic Self-ROM

Starting Position: Grasp affected arm just above the wrist, holding it on lap. Turn so the palm of the hand and wrist are facing up: (1) (supinated position).

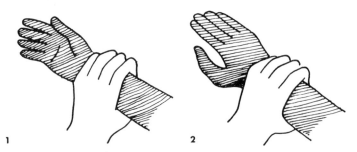

ROM: Turn in the opposite direction so the palm and wrist face down (2) (pronated position). Repeat movement.

ROM By Nurse

Wrist Flexion and Extension

Starting Position: Stabilize lower arm at the wrist with one hand. Hold the patient's fingers and hands with the other hand: (1), (2).

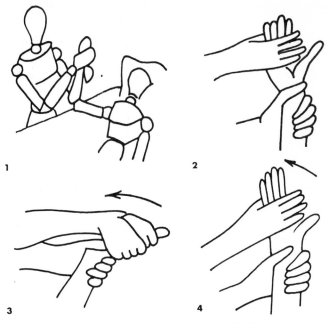

ROM: Bend wrist forward as far as it will go: (3). Then make a fist. Move hand backward as far as it will go, and then straighten fingers: (4). This produces ROM and stretching to both wrists and fingers as the muscles cross the wrist and finger joints. When a muscle bridges more than one joint, the muscle tends to tighten faster.

Hemiplegic Self-ROM

Starting Position: Interlock fingers of good and affected hands. Rest the affected wrist on the opposite knee.

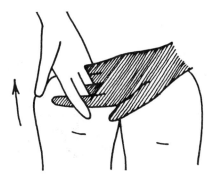

ROM: Bend affected hand up and down.

ROM By Nurse

Finger Flexion and Extension

Starting Position: Stabilize the hand by holding the palm of the hand in a neutral position.

ROM: Bend and straighten all fingers at one time.

If the fingers are stiff, bend and straighten each individual finger. To move each joint individually, stabilize directly below the joint to be moved.

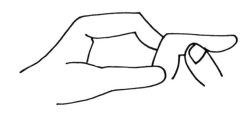

Hemiplegic Self-ROM

Starting Position: Place involved hand on lap or table, palm up.

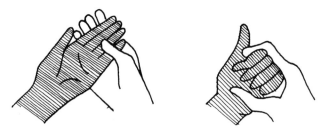

ROM: Straighten involved fingers, and then bend into a fist.

ROM By Nurse

Thumb Abduction

Starting Position: Stabilize the hand by holding the patient's fingers straight with one hand. Hold the thumb with the other: (1).

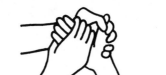

ROM: Pull the thumb away from the palm stretching the webbing between the thumb and index finger: (2).

Hemiplegic Self-ROM

Starting Position: Place involved hand on lap in neutral position, thumb and index finger facing up. Place thumb and index finger of uninvolved hand between the thumb web of the involved hand.

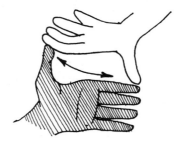

ROM: Spread thumb and index finger of uninvolved hand so thumb web of affected hand is spread open.

ROM By Nurse

Thumb Opposition

Starting Position: Same starting position as with thumb abduction: (1).

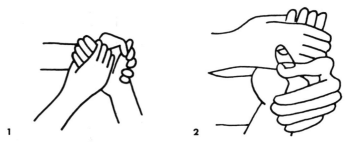

Move thumb over to the little finger describing a semicircle: (2).

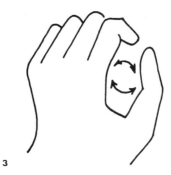

3

ROM: A good active exercise for this movement is for the patient to make circles between his thumb and each finger: (3).

Hemiplegic Self-ROM

Starting Position: Place involved hand on lap, palm up. Move thumb over to the little finger.

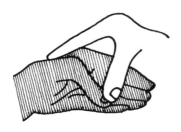

ROM By Nurse

Hip Flexion

Starting Position: Patient's leg flat on bed. Nurse holds under knee and under heel.

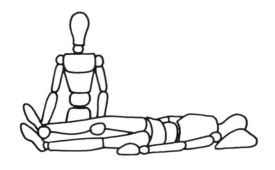

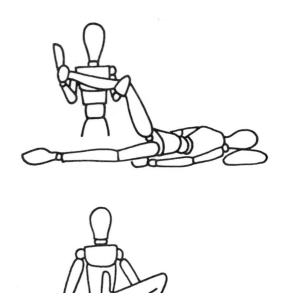

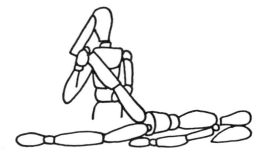

Raise knee toward chest producing as much bending at the hip as possible. Allow the knee to bend slightly or within the patient's tolerance and comfort.

Hamstring Stretching—Straight Leg Raising

[This is one of the problem areas where the muscle bridges two joints (hip and knee)].

Starting Position: Patient's leg flat on bed. Nurse holds under knee and heel.

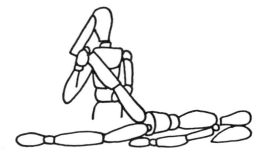

Keep the patient's leg straight. Gently lift leg up straight and as high as possible, hold for five count, lower the leg gently down to the bed, relax, and repeat. Move hands to hold the leg securely and comfortably.

Starting Position: Method 1   Bend hip up to 90° angle and bend the knee to 90°. Hold patient under knee and under heel: (1).

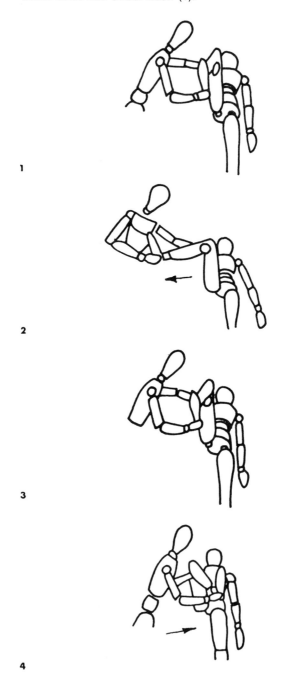

1

2

3

4

Keeping the hip and knee in place, turn the lower leg toward you, Step 2 (internal rotation of the hip), then turn it away from you, Step 4 (external rotation of the hip).

Starting Position: Method 2   Keep leg flat and in a "toes up" position on bed. Nurse places hands on top of patient's leg, one above the knee, one above the ankle.

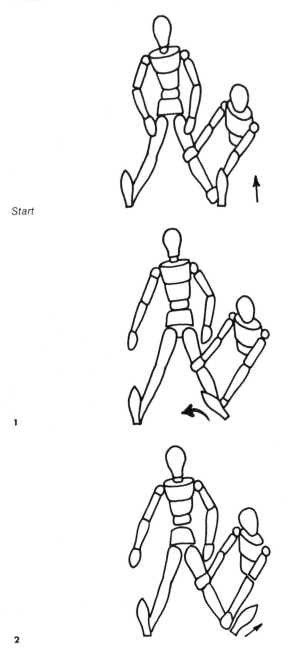

Start

1

2

Roll leg inward (Step 1—internal rotation)

Roll leg outward (Step 2—external rotation)

A patient can work actively on rotation using Method 2. Method 1 is very difficult done actively.

Abduction and Adduction of the Hip

Starting Position: Patient's leg flat on the bed. Your hand under the knee and under the heel: (1). Keep leg in toes up position.

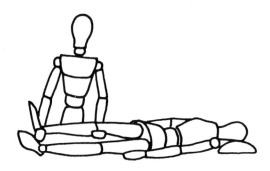

1

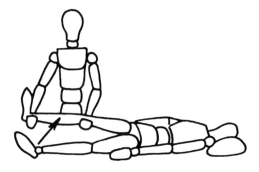

2

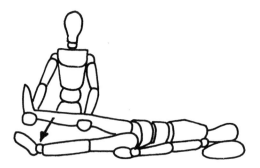

3

Keeping the leg flat on the bed pull the leg out toward you, (hip abduction) (2), then move the leg in toward the other leg (hip adduction: (3).

Knee Flexion and Extension

Starting Position: Method 1   Leg flat on bed. Nurse holds under patient's thigh and at the ankle as shown: (1).

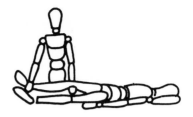

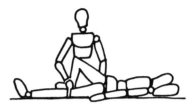

Lift the thigh and slide the heel along the bed toward the buttocks, causing flexion at the knee: (2). Pull out at heel, and rest leg straight on bed: (1). Repeat.

Method 2   Same starting position. Put thigh in approximately 90° of flexion, bend knee, straighten knee five times, then return to start position. Move hands to hold extremity securely and comfortably.

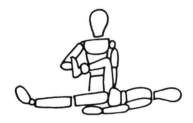

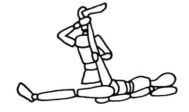

Dorsiflexion of Ankle (Heel Cord Stretch)

Starting Position: Patient's leg remains flat on the bed. Place one hand gripping heel as shown. Place other hand just above ankle, press downward toward the bed holding the leg flat.

Stand facing the bed with feet spread apart.

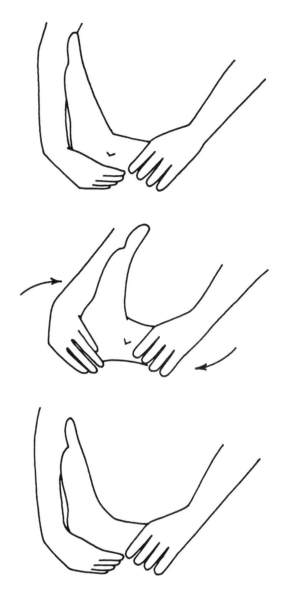

Pull down on heel, keep your elbow straight, and lean toward the head of the bed pressing your forearm against bottom of the patient's foot. This pushes the foot up toward the leg or bends the ankle and stretches the gastrocnemius muscle, or heel cord. Hold position firmly, count to five slowly, relax to the starting position, and repeat.

Inversion and Eversion of Foot

Starting Position: Patient's leg flat on bed. Put one hand on patient's leg to prevent internal or external movement of leg.

One hand holds foot as shown.

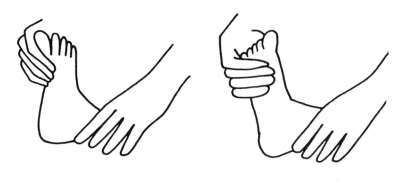

1   2

Turn foot outward (1).
Turn foot inward (2).

Toe Flexion and Extension

Starting Position: Hold foot as shown.

1

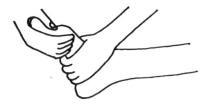

2

Bend all toes down: (1).
Pull all toes up: (2).

Flex and extend each toe joint individually if tightness or weakness of the toes has been determined (use the method described in ROM of the fingers).

This completes the ROM exercises. Remember to evaluate your patient and pick out the exercises needed. As we discuss how to accomplish different functional activities in the remainder of this book, evaluate each activity for the ROM it produces.

In summary:

1. Maintain a periodic check on your patient's range of motion. Do not let him get tight—it could retard or prevent his independence.
2. Do not overemphasize range of motion.
3. Do range of motion in conjunction with other activities.
4. Get your patient active as soon as possible.
5. Use passive ROM only as a starting point. Use ROM as a strengthening process quickly with active ROM and functional activities.

Now the patient is ready to move on his own to be taught some functional activities. The next three activities will be discussed in dialogue form. I strongly suggest that you try each activity yourself as you proceed through the instruction. Remember that players in our dialogues are the nurse and "Mr. Jones," the patient.

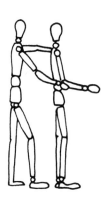

Moving Up and Down in Bed

The nurse prepares the scene by:

1. lifting the siderails,
2. rolling the bed flat,

3. turning down the blanket and straightening the sheets, and
4. checking Mr. Jones' pulse and any other cardiac symptoms.

The nurse:

> Mr. Jones, I will tell you how to move up further in bed so that you will be able to do it yourself. O.K.?

Mr. Jones:

> That's great! What do I do?

The nurse:

> Reach upward with your arms to hold onto the headboard. Bend your knees and hips, and place your feet flat on the bed. Now pull with your arms and push with your legs simultaneously. This will allow you to move up toward the head of the bed. There, you moved a little. Do it again. It might take you more than one try to get there. Now to move down in bed, Mr. Jones, just reverse the technique.

Check his pulse.

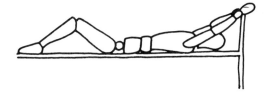

The patient can also reach for the edge of the mattress, the siderails, or a trapeze. Be sure he reaches above his head.

Or, the patient can get into a quarter-half sitting position and use his hand and elbows and arms to push (Figure 2-4).

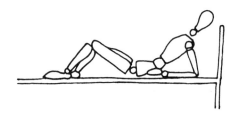

Find a bed and follow the nurse's instructions. Could you move up in bed according to these instructions? Remember to adapt techniques within the patient's limited physical abilities, e.g., a stroke patient would use only uninvolved upper and lower extremities. A hip fracture patient would *not* use the fractured hip unless it was approved for weight bearing.

To give assistance, hold the patient's feet so he can push easier with his leg or help the patient to move his buttocks by sliding your hands under his buttocks. Always be aware of your own body mechanics.

If the patient is not cooperative, keep working with him and encouraging him. This is difficult work for the patient, but as he becomes stronger it becomes easier for him. Furthermore, most patients become so pleased with their progress that they try harder.

- -

Test for Moving Up and Down in Bed

Try these questions to see if you learned how to move up in bed:

1. *Briefly, list step-by-step how to move up in bed.*
   a. _____
   b. _____
   c. _____
   d. _____
2. *To pull effectively with his arms the patient must reach* _____ *his head.*
3. *How does he move down in bed?* _____
4. *How would a hemiplegic move up in bed?* _____

Answers:
1. a. *Reach above head to headboard or use elbows to push.*
   b. *Bend knees.*
   c. *Push with feet and pull with arms simultaneously.*
   d. *Repeat until moved up into position.*
2. *Above.*
3. *Reverse the technique.*
4. *Follow same instructions, but use one arm and leg.*

- -

Moving Sideways in Bed

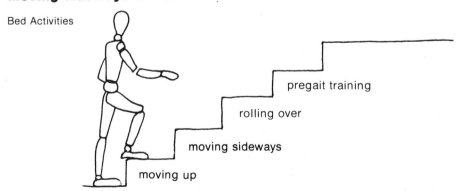

Bed Activities

pregait training

rolling over

moving sideways

moving up

Now that Mr. Jones can move up in bed he will use some of the techniques from that activity and learn to move sideways in bed. Let us say that Mr. Jones will be moving toward the right side of the bed. The nurse prepares the scene again by:

1. lifting the siderails,
2. rolling the bed flat,
3. turning down the blanket and straightening the sheets, and
4. checking Mr. Jones' pulse and any other cardiac symptoms.

The nurse:

First put your right hand on the siderail, Mr. Jones, just at the level of your shoulder. Don't reach too high.

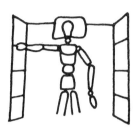

Now bend both of your knees, and put your feet flat on the bed. Lift up hips off the bed by pushing on your feet. Raise them just enough to clear the bed.

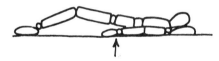

While you have your hips off the bed, shift your hips to the right, then put them down on the bed and relax. Now, move your head and shoulders over toward the right, scooting them is fine. You can pull with your arm, too, if necessary.
Good job, Mr. Jones.

Check his pulse.

A hemiplegic patient might have difficulty moving his involved leg in bed. To move it in bed, the patient should place his uninvolved foot under his involved ankle. He then lifts the involved leg just enough to clear the bed and moves his uninvolved leg as needed for the particular activity, thus moving his involved extremity. Likewise, the upper extremity is moved by the uninvolved upper extremity by grasping it at the wrist.

We sometimes call the activity of lifting up the buttocks, "bed pan" exercises. The patients seem to understand the movements better with a picture of the bed pan routine in their minds. To assist a patient with this activity, you can do any one or a combination of the following:

1. Hold his knees and feet in the flexed position.
2. Give him assistance to clear his buttocks off the bed. Do this by sliding your hand under the buttocks.
3. In conjunction with (2), give him assistance in shifting his hips to the side. Stand on the same side toward which he is moving. After putting your arm or arms under his buttocks, pull toward you.

Notice the motions necessary to move sideways in bed, and see the strengthening process in action. Briefly, bending hips and knees into position strengthens hip flexor muscles and hamstrings; raising the hips off the bed strengthens the buttocks, back, and abdominal muscles; and pulling with the arms strengthens hand and many arm muscles, especially the biceps. Each functional activity described in this chapter, when analyzed, strengthens particular muscle groups.

Find a bed and follow the nurse's instructions. Could you move over in bed according to these instructions?

Test for Moving Sideways in Bed

After you practice, please answer these questions:

1. *List briefly, step by step, how to move over in bed.*
   a. _____
   b. _____
   c. _____
   d. _____
   e. _____

2. How does a hemiplegic patient move his involved leg sideways? _____
_____

3. What are bed pan exercises?_____
_____

Answers:

1. *You moved sideways in bed if you,*
   a. *Put your hand on the siderail at shoulder level.*
   b. *Bent your knees.*
   c. *Lifted hips off bed.*
   d. *Shifted hips sideways.*
   e. *Pulled shoulder over.*
2. *By putting his uninvolved foot under his involved ankle.*
3. *Lifting the hips off the bed.*

Rolling Over in Bed

Bed Activities

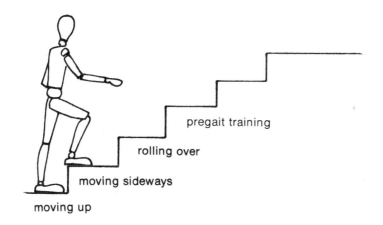

pregait training

rolling over

moving sideways

moving up

Preparations for this activity are the same as those for the two previous activities. *Remember* to check the pulse. The nurse stands on the *left side* of the bed. Mr. Jones is lying on his back.

The nurse:

Mr. Jones, I will want you to roll over on to your right side. (See illustration on p. 62.) You are lying in the middle of the bed now. Please move sideways toward me (to the left) so you'll have more room to roll over in the bed. Move just a little off center. Now cross your left leg over your right leg as far as possible. Cross your left arm over your chest and reach for the siderail or mattress. You can also hold onto the mattress or railing with your right arm, if you wish. Pull with your arms and roll over. Good job!

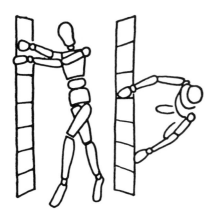

Check his pulse.

Crossing the "left leg over the right leg" as far as possible shifts the buttocks toward the right and starts the patient into the roll. If the patient is a hemiplegic and you are rolling him, put the good foot under the bad ankle to cross the legs. (See how many activities have this same motion? Your patients should learn this activity early.)

Sometimes the patient cannot roll over. In that case, try having him swing his arm and/or his leg across. This will create some momentum, which will help. (Notice that we are using the patient's body mechanics here. The heaviest part of a patient is his hips. By crossing his leg and arm in the direction to be turned, they are used as lever arms to lift the hip weight.)

Assistance might be needed when the patient first starts the activity, but as he does it he will become stronger; and it will be easier to do.

Find a bed and follow the nurse's instructions. Could you roll over in bed according to these instructions?

Test for Rolling Over in Bed

Please answer the following questions.

1. *List briefly, step-by-step, how to roll over in bed.*
    a. _____
    b. _____
    c. _____
    d. _____
2. *How are the patient's body mechanics used to help him roll over in bed?* _____
   _____
3. *If you are rolling to the left, which leg is crossed over the top of the other?* _____

Answers:

1. a. *Move off the center in bed.*
    b. *Cross your leg in the direction you are going—left over right.*
    c. *Cross your left arm across your chest and reach for the siderail.*
    d. *Pull over.*
2. *By using his legs as lever arms to shift the weight of his hips.*
3. *Right over left.*

How did you do? If you answered all questions correctly, you are doing fine. Let's continue.

We have now discussed all activities performed in bed. We've determined that Mr. Jones has some mobility. He's rather easy to handle in bed now, as he is able to help himself.

Special Note: A nurse can teach Mr. Jones these activities *during the course of the day* while giving him general nursing care. She taught him to move up in bed when he slid down too far, and she taught him to roll over while changing his sheets. Many hours are saved after a patient is taught to do these activities himself. After he learns, he does not need to ring the bell again to be moved in bed, he can do it alone. Your Mr. Jones can learn too!

Posttest

To check your understanding of this unit, please complete the following posttest. Write your answers in the space provided.

1. In which muscle groups is limitation of range of motion most likely to occur? ___
   _____

2. Range of motion activities accomplish two things. Name them.
   a. _____
   b. _____

3. Describe two different methods of using the arms to move up in bed.
   a. _____
   b. _____

4. Mrs. Smith has a broken right hip. What steps would she take to move toward the left side of the bed?
   a. _____
   b. _____
   c. _____
   d. _____
   e. _____
   f. _____

5. In which two joints might tightness occur if pillows were placed under the knees?
   a. _____
   b. _____

6. How does a hemiplegic or a hip fracture patient move his involved leg in bed?_____
   _____

7. Your patient is bedbound and unconscious. You have tested him for range of motion and have found that all joints except the ankle are limber. How would you proceed with range of motion activities?
   _____
   _____

8. Why is it important to use good bed positioning with your bedbound patient? ___
   _____

Now that you have answered these questions, compare your responses with those given below.
Answers:

1. Ones that bridge 2 or more joints, i.e., gastrocnemius, hamstrings, finger flexors.
2. Limber muscles and joints; start of strengthening.

3. a. Pull on headboard, mattress, trapeze.
   b. Quarter to half sitting position and push with arms.
4. a. Put left hand on siderail at shoulder level.
   b. Bent left knee.
   c. Lifted hips up off bed.
   d. Shifted hips to the left.
   e. Pulled shoulders over.
   f. Moved right leg over sideways.
5. a. Hips.
   b. Knees.
6. Puts the foot of the uninvolved leg under the ankle of the involved leg, lifts the leg slightly, and moves it with the uninvolved leg.
7. Position him properly. Do passive ROM along with bathing. Do passive ROM on ankle whenever in the room with patient.
8. To prevent deformities that might prevent patient independence later.

If you answered
   Eight correct, a perfect score!! Turn to next page.
   Seven correct, you are doing great!! Turn to next page.
   Five or six correct, this is satisfactory, but please look up and review your errors in the text before turning the page.
   Zero to four correct, sorry, poor score, please review the Bed Activities Section.

What else can Mr. Jones learn to do independently? Have you observed that each functional activity employs some action that the patient has learned in a previous activity? That's Progressive Mobilization—the Independence Staircase.

Pregait Training

This unit is called Pregait Training. Let's watch Mr. Jones learn to *sit up* and *stand up*.

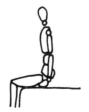 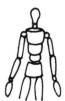

Assuming A Sitting Position

Mr. Jones is going to sit at the edge of the bed. Here, even more than with bed activities, it is important to check for cardiac symptoms and pulse responses. Dizziness is probably the most common occurrence when the patient first sits up.

Doctor S. orders "Dangling 5 minutes 2 X daily." Let's see how the nurse and Mr. Jones handle this one. The nurse prepares the scene by doing the following:

1. rolls the bed flat,
2. stands at the right side of the bed,
3. takes Mr. Jones' pulse, and
4. checks that he is wearing his shoes.

The nurse:

O.K., Mr. Jones, you have learned to move easily in bed. Now put together all those things you have learned and move to a sitting position at the edge of the bed. First, move sideways toward this edge of the bed. Roll over onto your right side. Good. Now slide your right arm underneath you with your elbow bent. That's tough. Maybe I can help you get it back there. You see you'll have to use it to push with in a minute. (1)

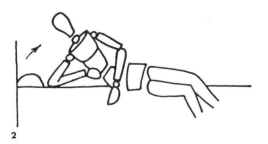

1

Now do these two things at the same time Drop your legs off the bed and start pushing up with your right elbow: (2)

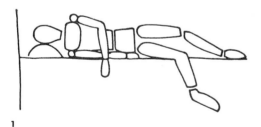

2

When the weight is on the right elbow, shift your weight to your right hand: (3)

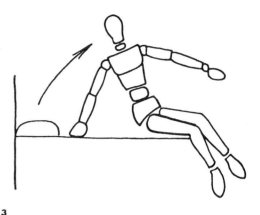

3

and keep pushing until you are upright: (4).

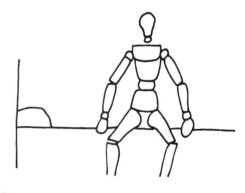

4

That's it. Are you dizzy? Your pulse is good.

A stroke patient should always roll onto his uninvolved side to sit up. It is much easier for him that way.

If the patient needs help, assist him as necessary but encourage him to do as much as he can alone. Three varying degrees of assistance might be as follows:

1. Help him move his legs off the bed.
2. Place your hand under his head, and help push his body up.
3. Put your arm under his shoulder, and help push him up to a sitting position.

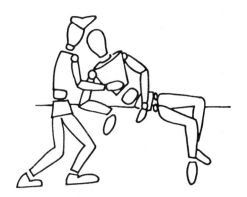

As soon as the doctor states that it is all right to have your patient sit, refer to sitting tolerance schedule (Table 2-1). If the patient cannot do any of this alone, do it all for him— just get him to sit!

Be sure to watch your body mechanics. Notice the difference between this method of assisting Mr. Jones and the method used by the nurse and Mr. Smith in the Body Mechanics section. This is *the correct* way to sit up even the largest or most involved patient.

You should now be concerned immediately with the next activity, sitting balance, but we will pause and check to see if you understand the sitting up procedure.

Practice: Find a bed and follow the nurse's instructions. Could you sit up according to these instructions?

1. *Briefly, list step-by-step how to sit at the edge of the bed.*
   a. _____
   b. _____
   c. _____
   d. _____
   e. _____
2. *If the patient needs help where would you assist him?* _____
   _____
3. *What is the most common occurrence when the patient sits up for the first time?*
   _____
4. *Which way should a stroke patient roll to get into a sitting position?* _____

Answers:

1. a. *Move toward edge of the bed.*
   b. *Roll onto your side.*

   c. *Put your arm underneath you.*
   d. *Drop legs off bed and push up with arms at the same time.*
   e. *Push until sitting.*
2. *At his legs, head, or shoulders.*
3. *The patient gets dizzy (blood pressure drops).*
4. *Onto his uninvolved side.*

If you feel that you can do this activity, go on to the next discussion.

Sitting Balance

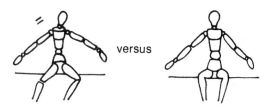

versus

When the patient is in a sitting position, it is important that he have good sitting balance. This means that he should be able to sit unsupported, even against resistance.

Have you ever had a patient who kept falling over when he sat on the edge of the bed? This is called poor sitting balance. To help him achieve good sitting balance, two factors must be considered: (1) good position of his body, and (2) practice.

Position: The patient should

1. sit level on the bed—bed flat—weight even on both buttocks;
2. position feet flat on the floor—wide base of support—shoes on (notice the principle of body mechanics here);
3. place arm, or arms, where he can push on them to hold him in a good, erect position. Initially, you may have to let him hold onto the edge of the bed to keep his balance, or you must assist him.

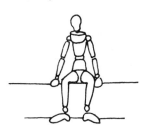

Practice: To work with him stand in front of him. By doing this you can help him move his hands or body as needed and can demonstrate what an upright position looks like. Also, in this position, you would not be tilting the bed with your own weight. (Did you ever sit on a bed and find yourself sliding toward the person near you who weighed more than you?) Give the patient all the advantage you can.

As the patient's sitting balance improves, he should be able to sit without holding onto the edge of the bed and should be able to move his arms around at will. He should practice reaching above his head, out to the side, out in front, etc. The patient should start by lifting his arms just a little and putting them back on the bed. Next time, he should raise them higher until he can do all the reaching activities easily and still maintain an erect position.

A patient with poor sitting balance will forever be slumped over in a wheelchair. (See also Chapter 6 for obtaining good sitting balance in a wheelchair.)

A good time to practice sitting balance is when the doctor first prescribes "dangling." If you consider the patient's sitting balance when he dangles, his dangling experience will be much more pleasurable.

Another important aspect of dangling is that it is the start of the "push" to build up your patient's sitting tolerance or his ability to stay out of bed for long periods of time (eventually all day). See again the Sitting Tolerance Schedule (Table 2-1). The more your patient is out of bed, the more opportunities he has to do different activities; and he will become stronger and more independent.

Can you see your patient climbing the Independence Staircase?

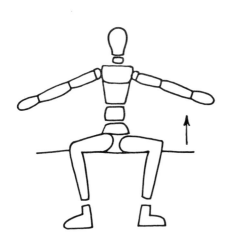

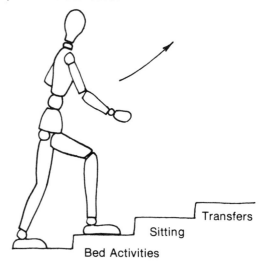

After he can do the above, the nurse should add resistance to the activity by pushing on the patient from either side, from the front or from the back. (Let the patient know that you are going to do this exercise so he does not think you are just trying to push him over!) Good sitting balance is achieved when the patient can do all this. This achievement means that the patient has *good trunk control.* Often, much time must be spent sitting with the patient to achieve good sitting balance. It is very important to spend the time because, if the patient does not have enough trunk control to sit, he will not have enough trunk control to stand.

Transfers

Your patient has come up quite far now on the Independence Staircase. This next step, transfers, is a difficult one. Often this is the highest level to which a patient can advance. If a patient can be independent at this level, he can function quite well in a home situation. He can cook, get around, get in and out of bed, get to the bathroom, etc. He is wheelchair independent. Acceptance of such a goal should not be considered "giving up." It is a reasonable alternative for the person who cannot be expected to walk functionally. Individuals commonly live independently at home, work at demanding professions, travel, and engage in sports—all from a wheelchair. Such a person accepts no limitations on his horizons. With that in mind, independence in transferring is a *big step*, and we want Mr. Jones to learn how to move from his bed to a wheelchair.

Standing Transfers

Standing transfers in all situations, i.e., bed, toilet, regular chair, or car, are accomplished in basically the same manner as bed to wheelchair. The variations depend only on structural differences in the appliances. Set the scene by doing the following:

1. Roll the bed flat and check Mr. Jones' pulse rate. Then Mr. Jones sits up. His sitting balance is good. Pulse is stable.
2. Adjust the height of the bed so Mr. Jones' feet will touch the floor when he sits on the edge of the bed.
3. Put on his shoes. This is done so Mr. Jones has a good solid foundation. You do not want your patients to slip. If they do not have shoes on, have them transfer barefooted rather than wearing "slick" slippers. Do not transfer patients with just elastic stockings on their feet. They will certainly slip.
4. Bring in the wheelchair, and check to see that it is a safe chair: good framework, brakes lock well, foot plates work properly, and it wheels easily. The wheelchair in this case is a standard wheelchair. (See Chapter 6 for fitting particular patients.)
5. Determine which side is Mr. Jones' strongest side. It is determined that *Mr. Jones is strongest on the left*. If the chair is placed on the patient's strongest side, the patient will have more confidence and find it easier to transfer.
6. Lift up the foot plates, removing obstacles that are in the way.
7. Place the chair on his left side, parallel to the bed, and in a position where the raised foot plates are between Mr. Jones' feet and the bed.
8. *Lock* the brakes! This is so the chair will not roll when he puts his weight on it.

9. Stand in front of Mr. Jones, near enough to help, but do not hinder his movements.

Remember body mechanics, of course. Be prepared. Now Mr. Jones is ready to move from his bed to the wheelchair.

The nurse:

Mr. Jones, slide forward to the edge of the bed. Place your right hand flat on the bed and your left hand on the right arm rest of the chair: (1).

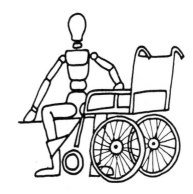

1

Now lean forward slightly at the hips. Push on your hands, straighten your legs and trunk, and stand up: (2).

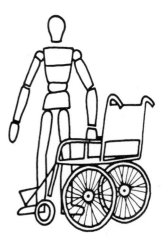

2

Now start moving your feet toward the left. First left foot, then right, turning them so you being moving in a circle. Use small steps. Move your left hand to the other arm rest. Keep turning until you are standing directly in front of the chair and feel the back of both legs against the chair. Put your right hand on the chair, too. (3).

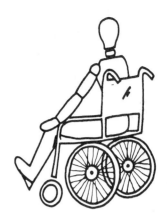

4

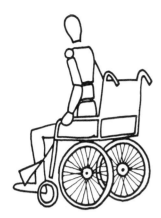

3

Lean forward slightly, and sit down slowly. Lower yourself with your arms and legs. Slide back in the chair and sit squarely: (4).

Put your feet on the foot plates. Good, you're there, safe and sound! To get back to bed, Mr. Jones, you would reverse the process, placing the chair again so that you would be moving toward your good side.

His pulse is fine. He has responded well to the activity.

When Mr. Jones leans slightly forward before he stands, this movement centers his weight over his feet. Put your hands on Mr. Jones' rib cage to help him stand if needed. Your knees should be bent, back straight. Brace his leg or legs with your legs if he needs it. As Mr. Jones gets stronger, you will have to help him less and less. He will reach a point where you can stand farther away from him while he does the activity alone. Remember, DO NOT give assistance unless needed.

If the patient is a stroke patient with no responses at all in the hemiplegic side, or if the patient is a nonweight-bearing patient on one side, he should pivot on the uninvolved foot.

Now you practice. 1. as if you were Mr. Jones and 2. the nurse.

Test for Standing Transfers

Answer these questions.

1. *Where does the patient push to stand up?* _____
2. *How does a stroke patient turn in a circle?* _____
   _____
3. *Where does the nurse hold Mr. Jones to assist him?* _____
   _____
4. *How should the wheelchair be placed in relation to*
   Mr. Jones: _____
   the bed: _____
5. *Name two safety factors regarding the wheelchair that are important for patient transfers:*
   a. _____
   b. _____

Answers:

1. *On the arm rest of the chair and on the bed.*
2. *He pivots on his uninvolved leg.*
3. *Around the rib cage area. You should never pull up the patient's arm; this could cause damage especially to a hemiplegic arm.*
4. *a. On his stronger side.*
   b. Parallel to the bed—between the bed and Mr. Jones' feet.
5. *a. Lock brakes.*
   b. Raise foot plates.

If you answered these correctly you are doing well. Transfers done properly are very important to you and your patient. Be sure that you can do the standing transfer step-by-step and feel comfortable with the dialogue so you will be able to teach a patient.

Sliding Board Transfers

If your patient cannot stand, sliding board transfers are ideal. This particular transfer serves well the paraplegic or quadriplegic patient or anyone who for some reason cannot stand to do a standing transfer. I have used it with patients who have had severe knee flexion contractures and hemiplegic patients who are too heavy or weak for me to assist to a standing position. This transfer is ideal for families when they are without the aid of a nurse or therapist.

To do this transfer, one first must have a wheelchair with removable arms (refer to Chapter 6 regarding removable arms) and a sliding board. Sliding boards are now standard rehabilitation items and can be purchased from most medical supply offices. If one needs to be manufactured, a board made of a strong wood, 10 inches x 28 inches, and varnished heavily, will work well.

Position the wheelchair as with a standing transfer. Lock the brakes, remove the foot rest closest to the bed if possible, or lift up the foot plate. Remove the arm of the wheelchair closest to the bed. The patient is sitting at the edge of the bed. He should be wearing shoes, and his feet should be touching the floor. Because bare skin sticks, the patient should also be wearing slacks or pajamas so he can slip easily on the sliding board. Direct the patient to lean over to the side away from the wheelchair, and put one end of sliding board under his buttocks. Put the other end of the sliding board on the chair seat.

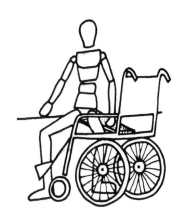

Stand in front of the patient. Block his knees with your knees, and put your hands around his trunk or use a belt around his waist to balance him. Direct him to lean forward slightly. He should then push with his arms, lift his buttocks slightly off the board, and slide over toward the wheelchair. Encourage the patient to use all the muscle strength he has present, both in his legs and in his arms. You might need only to pull on his belt to help him. Repeat this action until the transfer is completed. Allow the patient to place his hands along the sliding board, or wherever he can on the wheelchair to move himself most effectively. Many patients can learn to do this transfer independently, especially the paraplegic patient.

If the patient cannot help at all, you might need to press against his knees and pull him forward toward you, creating a rocking movement that will allow you to slide him sideways on the board and into the wheelchair. Always remember your body mechanics.

If you do not have a sliding board, a pillow can be placed over the wheelchair tire to span the gap between the bed and the wheelchair and protect the patient from the wheelchair parts. Then a transfer similar to a sliding board transfer can be performed.

Using a pillow to transfer is more difficult than using the sliding board because the sliding feature of the board is eliminated and the patient must lift his hips up enough to shift his buttocks sideways toward the wheelchair. Though this method is more difficult, it is possible to perform and is safer for the patient and nurse than standing a person unable to stand. Also, considering the patient who *can* lift his buttocks up easily and shift his hips but cannot stand, this method works well. If he can use a pillow, a sliding board is not needed.

After the patient can move easily across to the chair, he can often discard pillows *and* sliding boards and lift himself across into the chair.

Test for Sliding Board Transfers

Please answer the following questions to test your understanding of sliding board transfers.

1. Describe the type of wheelchair needed to perform a sliding board transfer. _____
   _____

2. Name two reasons for using a pillow for this type of transfer. _____
   _____
   _____

3. Does a patient have to be able to lift his hips to use a sliding board? _____
   Why?_____
   _____

4. What type of patient would use a sliding board?_____
   _____

Answers:

1. *Removable arms—preferably removable legs.*
2. *a. Spans the gap between the wheelchair and the bed.*
   b. Protects the patient from the wheelchair parts.
   c. Eliminates the need for purchasing a sliding board if the patient can initially use this method or if he can be progressed from using a sliding board to using this method.
3. *No. You can pull him over on the sliding board, or use a rocking motion to slide him over.*
4. *One who could not come to a standing position due to paraplegia, quadriplegia, weakness, weight, or the limited strength of the assistant.*

Did you answer the questions correctly?

NOTE: You have just learned a number of different transfers. It is important to evaluate your patient carefully to decide which method to use. Always choose the method most appropriate for the patient at the time. As the patient progresses with his rehabilitation, the method of transferring him should be changed accordingly.

Continue now to teach Mr. Jones how to use a wheelchair.

Wheelchair Ambulation and Weight Shifting

Wheelchair Ambulation

The nurse: "Unlock the brakes, Mr. Jones. There are two. When unlocked the brakes do not touch the wheels. (You might need to teach your patient to do this. Refer to Chapter 6 regarding wheelchair brakes.)

Place your hands on the steel rims and push forward and evenly on both wheels. The wheelchair will move straight forward.

To turn to the left, push only on the right wheel. To turn to the right, push only on the left wheel.

To go backward, pull evenly on both wheels."

If the patient is a stroke patient and has function only on one side, he must use his arm and leg on the one side to wheel his chair. This is accomplished in the following manner:

1. raise the foot plate on the uninvolved side, and place the patient's foot on the floor (with shoes on),
2. put the uninvolved hand on the wheel, and
3. push as above with the one hand and "pull" with the foot.

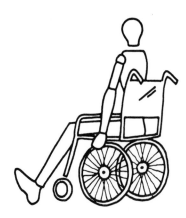

"Pulling" with the foot is done by extending the knee, placing the heel of the foot down firmly on the ground, keeping it on the ground, and forcibly flexing the knee. The patient can "pull" the chair along in this manner. (Sometimes patients use their toes to pull.) Likewise, the foot acts as a rudder to straighten the chair out as one goes along. Because of the use of the foot, it is very important for this particular type patient to be in a chair which allows his whole foot to touch the floor easily. (See Chapter 6 regarding hemi wheelchairs.) If the foot does not touch the floor, the patient cannot wheel the chair.

MAJOR SAFETY NOTE regarding wheelchairs: Always lock the brakes and raise the foot plates when the chair has stopped and the patient intends to get out of it.

Weight Shifting in the Wheelchair

It is important that patients be able to shift their weight in the wheelchair for two reasons:

1. Pressure must be taken off the buttocks to prevent decubiti from prolonged sitting. (A patient should shift his weight at least every fifteen minutes. See also Chapter 9.)
2. The patient must be able to lift his buttocks so he can reposition himself in the chair.

Wheelchair Exercise

Wheelchair push-ups is an exercise designed to accomplish the above mentioned points as well as to strengthen the patient's arms. Wheelchair push-ups in the true sense is an exercise for the paraplegic patient who has absolutely no sensation in his buttocks area.

Repeating the push-up ten to fifty times at one session strengthens the patient's triceps and shoulder depressors, which are particularly necessary for crutch gait. Obviously the exercise would be good for any patient you are teaching to crutch walk or walk with a walker.

Method:

Place one hand on each arm rest, elbows bent. Keep the shoulders level, lean forward slightly, push on the hand and straighten the elbows, lifting the hips off of the chair. Hold to count of five.

Holding the hips off the chair allows the circulation to flow freely in the buttocks and the patient's position in the chair to be changed.

A hemiplegic patient also must be able to shift his weight in the chair, but because of the lack of use of one side of his body a wheelchair push-up is impossible. However a modified push-up can be done. Method:

Use one hand on the arm rest.

Place feet on the foot plates.

Lean forward slightly, bending at the hips. (Do not lean so far forward as to fall out of the chair or tip it over).

Push with arm and both legs as much as possible to lift the hips.

Note: If you have a patient who continually slips down in the wheelchair, this is what you can do to help him get back into position:

1. Stand in front of him and put his feet on the foot plates. Pulling his trunk toward you, bend him at the hips. Have him push with his hands or one hand and with his legs. As he is pushing, you push against his knees. He will slide back in the chair.
2. Have him sit on a towel in the wheelchair. You stand behind the wheelchair. Position the patient forward (bend him at the hips). Hold onto the towel and pull it toward you. This will pull his buttocks back in the chair.

To move a patient in a wheelchair successfully the main point to remember is to *have him lean forward.* To prevent the patient from sliding out of the wheelchair keep his hips in a flexed position and his buttocks at the back of the wheelchair. A method used to accomplish this when standard restraints do not work is to fold a sheet in half, with the end of it hanging through the back of the chair. Place a rolled pillow on the front of the chair on top of the sheet. Wrap the rest of the sheet firmly *over* the pillow and put the end of the sheet through the back of the chair. Tie the ends of the sheet to the wheelchair (Figure 2-7). Lift the patient into the wheelchair so that his knees rest on the pillow and the patient's buttocks are against the back of the chair.

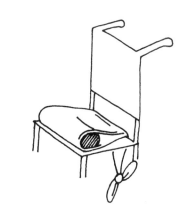

Figure 2-7   Moving a Wheelchair Patient

Test for Wheelchair Ambulation and Weight Shifting

Please answer the following questions about wheelchairs:

1. *If you want the wheelchair to turn to the right, which wheel do you push?*_____
2. *How do you know that the brakes are locked?*_____
_____

3. *What is the most important point to remember when fitting a hemiplegic with a wheelchair?*
_____

4. *What are two ways wheelchair push-ups can help patients.*
   a. _____
   b. _____
5. *What is the main point to remember to reposition a patient in a wheelchair?*_____
_____

Answers:

1. *The left wheel.*
2. *When the brake touches the wheel and the wheels do NOT move!*
3. *That his foot touches the floor. Otherwise he will not be able to use his one hand and one foot to push the chair.*
4. *If you answered any of the following you were correct:*
   a. *Prevent decubiti by weight shifting.*
   b. *Slide back in chair.*
   c. *Strengthening arms.*
5. *Direct the patient to lean forward.*

Please review if you were unsure about any of the answers. Otherwise, continue.

Standing

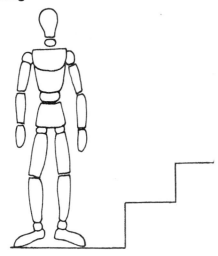

Stand-Ups

Transfers and standing activities go hand-in-hand. As the patient's standing (both strength and balance) improves, his transfers get better; and as his transfers get better, his standing improves.

Practically speaking, we can transfer someone out of bed who cannot stand alone because we help them as much as they need to be helped. If we do it in the manner discussed in the transfer section, the patients learn to help themselves in the process. You can help them control their trunk and legs. However, for patients to progress to independent transfers and to walking, they must be taught to stand and balance themselves. Even if a patient cannot walk, the ability to stand is still extremely helpful as it will enable standing transfers, pulling up pants, toileting, reaching, and numerous other functions. Recall that earlier we said that if a person could lift ten pounds with his leg muscles but could not stand up from a chair he was stuck. Therefore, the purpose of this exercise becomes obvious. We will now discuss exercises to increase stand-up ability, strength, and balance.

The exercise is called "stand-ups." It is as simple as it sounds. The instruction to the patient to get him to perform the exercise is

"stand up." The act of standing up is remarkable in what it accomplishes. When you stand up, you are strengthening every muscle in your body to a certain degree. You use your legs and their muscles to get up and you use your trunk muscles to retain a good, erect position. The main accomplishment is in the strengthening achieved in the thigh muscles (especially the quadriceps). The exercise is also a general conditioning program for the heart, lungs, and autonomic reflexes that maintain the blood flow to the head. Standing is very important to the patient's later ability to walk.

The equipment needed for this exercise includes (1) a chair, (2) a table, (3) some books, firm pillows, or pieces of wood to build up the height of the chair, (4) Mr. Jones (the patient), and (5) the nurse (an assistant), or anyone who wants to help the patient.

More than any other exercise, this exercise utilizes the psychological need of the patient to be encouraged and to be successful. Success breeds success. Stand-ups, if done correctly, can produce high patient motivation and independence. This is accomplished by adjusting the exercise equipment so the patient *can* get into the standing position *alone*. By being able to accomplish an activity alone, the patient feels successful, is motivated and is encouraged. The stand-ups are performed this way:

1. Raise the height of a chair seat with pillows, phone books, newspapers, etc.

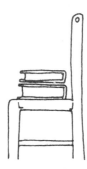

2. Estimate the height of the chair needed to allow the patient to stand alone. A good height at which to start can be determined by measuring the patient's leg from the knee to the foot and making the chair height one and a half times that

length, e.g., patient's leg measures 18 inches from the knee to the foot—one and a half times that amount is 27 inches—start with a chair approximately 27 inches high (floor to seat). The angle of the knee will be approximately 130°.

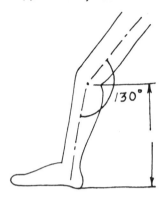

3. Sit the patient on this chair facing the table.

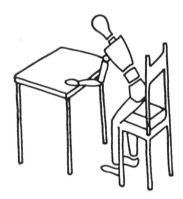

4. Check the patient's pulse.
5. Put the patient's hand, or hands, flat on the table.
6. Put his feet on the floor (shoes on). They should touch fairly well.
7. Patient should be sitting at the *edge* of the chair. If he sits too far back he will find it more difficult to get up (refer to transfers and body mechanics principles).
8. Have the patient lean forward slightly, push down with his hand slightly on the table, straighten his knees and back, and stand-up. Hands should be used mostly for balance. *The work should be done by the legs, not the arms.*

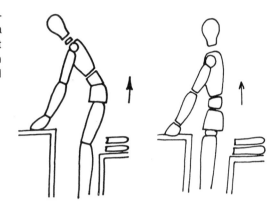

The patient should be able to *stand* alone, with *absolutely no* help from you.

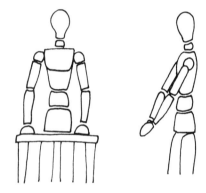

With this accomplishment, the patient is encouraged. He will be pleased with himself and ready to work harder. He now knows that *he* can stand up alone. He knows that *he* can succeed. With that important point accomplished, you can proceed with the exercise.

If you determine that at the initial starting height the activity was too easy for the patient, let him know that he is doing well, that the stand-up was too easy for him, and that you are going to lower the seat about an inch or so and he can try the exercise again. Keep lowering the seat until it is just moderately difficult for him to stand up alone. When you have found this level, the patient can begin the stand-up exercise. Repeat the exercise as follows: patient stands up—remains standing about ten seconds—sits slowly—sits about fifteen seconds; repeat the exercise ten to twenty times at one session. The number of repetitions should correspond to the patient's tolerance. Someone very weak would do less than ten repetitions. Later, as endurance increases, he could do as many as thirty. This exercise also builds endurance. The exercise should be done two to four times daily, spaced at even intervals, i.e., 9 a.m., 12 noon, 4 p.m. and 7 p.m. The more stand-ups he does, the stronger he becomes.

In a hospital, the bed can be raised to an appropriate height to do stand-ups effectively.

As the patient gains strength, the chair should be lowered gradually until the patient can stand from a regular chair by himself. He will then have strong legs.

We have found that strong legs are especially important with stroke patients or patients with hip fractures. Because of the added work put on the normal leg to compensate for the weak leg, it must be "super strong" to allow effective walking. We have seen this strengthening method work over and over again, for almost any condition that requires leg strengthening. It works primarily, we feel, because it is simple to do, has a strong motivating effect, and the instructions are simple to follow. The directions can be explained easily by demonstrations, gestures, or tactile assistance, which allows even very confused or aphasic patients to understand the exercise.

Standing Balance

During the standing phase of the stand-up, the patient should also practice standing balance. At first, he should keep his hands on the table for balance. Then, have him lift his hands off the table, raise them sideways and overhead while maintaining his balance. The patient's ability to complete this exercise will increase with practice and gradual increase of strength. Later, resistance can be given to the patient by pushing him unexpectedly from side to side, forward and back. This will stress his balance and will increase his ability. (See the section on sitting balance for this exercise.)

Extra Notes on Standing, Stand-Ups, and Standing Balance—

1. After strength, endurance, and balance are gained, the patient should be instructed to continue the exercise, at least daily, to maintain the strength in his legs.

2. If a patient has a fractured leg, use a block of wood under the *uninvolved* foot for him to stand on. This helps him keep his weight off the fracture.

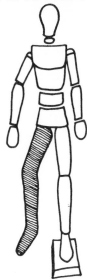

3. If a patient is too weak to perform the stand-up exercise alone, adjust the chair as high as possible and help him until he can stand alone.

4. To evaluate when a patient is able to stand, test his quadriceps strength. If he can hold against some resistance he can probably stand. Also, *just try* to stand him. If he can stand, it is obvious that he can perform the exercise. If he cannot, use the standard PRE exercises until his leg strength increases sufficiently to stand.

5. If the patient's balance is very bad, have him assume a wide base of support on the table with his hands.

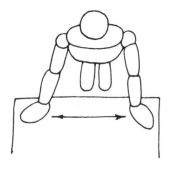

Now for some questions and practice regarding standing, stand-ups, and standing balance.

1. Place two to three books in a chair. Sit on them and place your hands on the table according to the stand-up exercises. Hold one foot off the floor. Stand up and sit down ten times. Now remove both books and repeat the same exercise. Which way was easier? Can you see that it is easier to stand up from a higher chair? _____

2. This is Mr. Jones' first attempt at stand-ups. How much would you elevate the chair? __
_____
_____
_____
_____

3. If Mr. Jones is having terrible standing balance problems, what could you do?
_____
_____

4. How many times a day should a patient do stand-ups to make the program effective?
_____
_____

5. What muscles are most strengthened by the stand-up exercises?
_____
_____

6. How long and how often should a patient continue these exercises after he goes home? _____
_____

7. Why are stand-ups so effective?
a. _____
_____
b. _____

8. What is the most important single goal of the stand-up program? _____
_____

Answers:

1. The second way should have been easier. Was it?
2. One and a half times his leg length from knee to foot, or, the amount needed that he be able to stand up alone.
3. Spread his hands apart on the table.
4. Two to four times a day. (Four would be better.)
5. Quadriceps and other thigh muscles.

6. At least once a day forever, if it is a stroke patient.
7. a. They are motivating to the patient.
   b. They are easy to do.
8. That the patient be able to stand up alone.

I realize that there was a great deal of information in this section. After answering the questions you may want to reread the information. This is a very important section, in that the stand-up exercise can be used with many different patients.

Stairclimbing

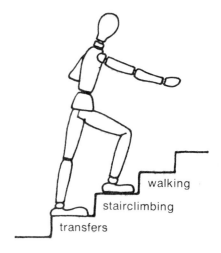

walking

stairclimbing

transfers

Stairclimbing

Stair Climbing, or "Up With the Good, Down With the Bad."

You might be surprised to find stairclimbing as our next step to independence. It would seem that stairclimbing should be taught after walking. (It should be taught last for a patient using crutches.) But for the hemiplegic patient or one with weak or uncoordinated legs used *before* walking, stairclimbing adds certain abilities.

Generally, stand-ups increase the strength of the quadriceps muscles and increase the ability to stand and balance. The exercise is done with both feet on the floor.

Generally, stairclimbing increases the strength of the individual quadriceps muscle and increases the ability to stand and balance while the body is in motion. Walking does not increase quadriceps strength as stairclimbing does. EMG studies *prove this true.* Using stairclimbing as an exercise, the patient:

1. learns to shift his weight when picking up his feet,
2. learns to place his feet properly,
3. learns to take small even steps,
4. gains additional strength in his legs, and
5. learns to maintain his balance when one leg is off the ground. (If he is a hemiplegic, stair climbing will improve his reflexes and the spasticity in the quadriceps muscle.)

Additionally, when you tell a patient that he is going to start moving his feet, looking up a flight of stairs is not as frightening as looking down a long hall. The eye to floor distance is much less on stairs than on the level.

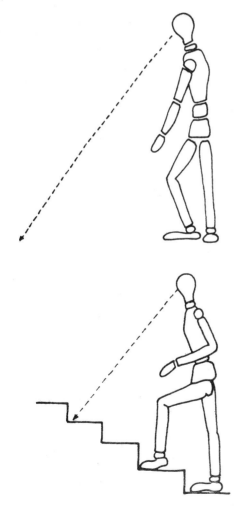

Usually our patients go down the stairs forward, but if frightened or very weak, walking down backward gives the patient the same "eye to floor" confidence, eliminates the turning procedure on the stairs, and places the involved hip in a more extended position to help facilitate the action of the gluteus maximus muscle.

In the Rehabilitation Center we use the stairs progressively, as we do stand-ups, by starting the patient on 2-inch stairs and advancing through 4-inch to 6-inch stairs as his strength and ability increase. This progression is good if the facilities are available, otherwise, you can use the normal stair (6-inch), foot stool, or curb and give more assistance, lessening the assistance as the patient improves.

It is always easier to teach stairclimbing by demonstrating it first. Now let's see how the nurse and Mr. Jones approach this exercise. The nurse sets the scene:

1. She uses a 6-inch staircase with a railing on both sides.
2. She wheels Mr. Jones up to the staircase in his wheelchair and locks the wheelchair.
3. She demonstrates stairclimbing to Mr. Jones.
5. She takes his pulse.

(The instructions here are for a patient with one involved leg, two good arms and use of two railings. A hemiplegic patient would only use the railing on his uninvolved side. Also, if only one railing were available, a person would use only one hand on that railing.)

Note: Good leg refers to the uninvolved or strong leg; *bad* leg refers to the involved or weak leg. In the drawings the solid foot represents the bad foot. The little saying "Up with the good foot, down with the bad" really helps patients remember how to climb stairs!

The nurse:

>Okay, Mr. Jones, now you will climb the stairs. Stand up from your chair. Push on the arm rests—don't pull on the railing.
>
>Stand up straight and get your balance.
>
>Good.

Going Up

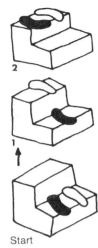

Start

Going Down

Start

Now place your hands on the railings. Keep your 'bad' leg straight. *Step up with your good leg first.* Place your foot totally on the chair. Now push on your hands (don't pull) and step up with your 'bad' leg to the same step. Get your foot all the way on the step and have your feet spread evenly.

Now get your balance.

Move your hands higher on the railing and repeat the same process for the next step. Take one step at a time until you arrive at the top of the stairs.

Turn around by taking small steps in a circle.

Stand facing down the steps with both feet close to the edge of the step. Place your hands on the railings slightly ahead of your feet. This is for balance. *Step down with your 'bad' leg first,* lowering your weight slowly with your 'good' leg.

(Feet should be about 6 inches apart.) Do you have your balance, Mr. Jones?

O.K., now quickly put your 'good' foot down beside your 'bad' foot.

Regain your balance again, and repeat the same process for each step.

Some patients' legs are about equal in strength and they can step one foot over another. This will aid in strengthening both legs. A hemiplegic patient should always go up and down stairs one at a time. When going down stairs, the patient should always lean slightly forward since the tendency is to fall backward, not forward. If the patient descends the stairs backwards, he should follow all instructions given, only step down backwards.

To assist the patient, you should be behind him when he is going up the stairs and be in front of him when he is going down. Use a wide base of support with one foot on each step. Be close enough to the patient to balance him if necessary or hold him if he starts to fall.

REMEMBER your body mechanics!

If you are working with a patient and he begins to fall, hold him as close to you as possible to help him rebalance himself. If it is evident that he cannot regain his balance and will fall, you should hold him close, keep your back straight, bend your knees, lower him to the floor, or, sit him down on the step.

Questions:

1. *A hemiplegic patient should climb _____ stairs at a time.*
2. *Coming down the steps, the patient should position himself so that both of his feet are _____ to the edge of the step.*
3. *The patient should always keep his hands _____ of his feet for balance.*
4. *The patient should step up with his _____ foot first and down with his _____ foot.*
5. *For safety, when assisting a patient, you should be _____ him when going up the stairs and _____ of him when coming down the stairs.*
6. *Name two things which are accomplished by doing stairclimbing as an exercise.*
   a. _____
   b. _____

Answers:

1. *One.*
2. *Close.*
3. *Ahead.*
4. *Good or uninvolved; bad or involved.*
5. *Behind; ahead.*
6. *If you answered any two of these you were correct;*
   a. *learns to shift his weight,*
   b. *learns to place feet,*
   c. *gains strength in legs,*
   d. *learns to maintain balance when one foot is off the floor,*
   e. *learns to take small steps,*
   f. *develops quadriceps spasticity in hemiplegic patient.*

Now let's see what *stairclimbing with crutches* would look like.

The same method of stairclimbing would be used with a patient with a fractured leg or hip fracture who could not bear weight. In such a case, crutches would be used. Crutches are to be considered with the "bad" or involved foot.

Methods Using Crutches

Use of two crutches going up:

Step up with "good" or uninvolved leg first, then bring crutches and "bad" or involved leg up. Do not step on the involved leg.

Use of two crutches going down: Stand close to the edge of the step, put crutches down, and put "bad" or involved leg down, then quickly put the "good" or uninvolved leg down. Do not step on the involved leg.

Notice that crutches are spread apart enough for balance and are placed in the middle of the stair. A patient's balance will be better if he places the "bad" or involved foot on the step, but does not put weight on it. Stairclimbing can also be done in a non-weight-bearing fashion by using one crutch and the railing. Use the same method except that, when the second crutch would be moved, move the hand on the railing instead.

The "solid" foot represents the bad or involved foot

Two-Crutch Method

Going Up   Going Down

Start

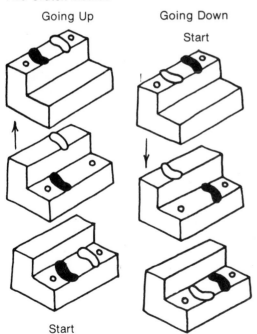

Start

Crutch-railing Method

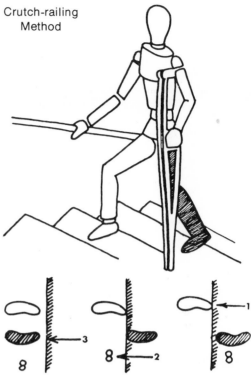

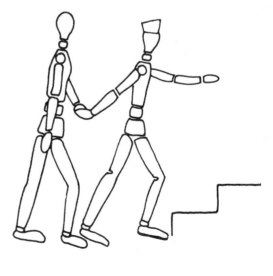

The nurse and Mr. Jones have climbed stairs. They are nearly to the top of the Independence Staircase. Before proceeding to the posttest for this unit, please reread the section "Where to Start Progressive Mobilization." Is it clearer? Please take the posttest on the following page to see if you will be able to take *your* Mr. Jones this far up the Independence Staircase!

Test for Pregait Training

Place your answers in the space provided.

1. Crutches are moved along with the _____ leg.
2. When stairclimbing, step up with the _____ leg first; and down with the _____ leg first.
3. It is important that a patient be able to stand alone during stand-ups. Why? _____
   _____
4. a. You have evaluated Mr. Jones and have decided that he has no muscle tightness, could move about in bed alone, and could get to sitting position alone. He has good sitting balance. He needed moderate assistance with transfers because he could not stand up easily from the bed. His knees buckled when he moved his feet. What exercises on the Independence Staircase would you use with Mr. Jones?
   _____
   _____

   b. Would you walk him at this point? _____
5. Describe how a patient gets to a sitting position at the edge of the bed.
   _____
   _____
   _____
6. If Mr. Jones has a weak left side, on which side of him would you position the wheelchair for a transfer? _____
   Why? _____
7. When a patient gets in or out of a wheelchair, what is the most important factor to remember? _____
   _____
8. What is the most important factor to consider about a wheelchair if a stroke patient is to wheel himself? _____
   _____
9. Stairclimbing accomplishes five goals. Name two.
   a. _____
   b. _____
10. Describe briefly how you would proceed with stand-up exercises. (Name equipment and method in your answer.) _____
    _____
    _____
    _____
    _____
    _____
11. What muscle groups strengthen most with the stand-up exercise?
    _____
12. Mr. Smith has considerable weakness in the muscles on his involved side. He has poor trunk control. When he sits he leans toward his involved side. What exercise do you use to correct this? _____
    _____

Now that you have answered these questions, compare your responses with those given here and on the following page.

Answers:

1. *Bad or involved leg.*
2. *Good or uninvolved leg; bad or involved leg.*

3. It encourages and motivates him. It makes him feel successful—remember "success breeds success."
4. a. Transfer training, stand-up exercises.
   b. No, because you should strengthen his legs first.
5. a. Move toward edge of bed.
   b. Roll onto side.
   c. Put arm underneath.
   d. Drop legs off bed and push up with arms at same time. ·
   e. Push until sitting.
6. Right side; so he can move toward his good side.
7. Lock the brakes!
8. The wheelchair must be low enough so the patient's feet can touch the floor.
9. If you named any two of these you were correct.
   The patient:
   a. learns to shift weight,
   b. learns to maintain balance on one foot,
   c. learns to place feet properly,
   d. teaches himself to take small even steps,
   e. gains additional strength. (Improves reflexes and spasticity in the quadriceps muscle for the stroke patient.)
10. Use chair with books, etc. to elevate it. Place in front of a table. Elevate chair so patient can stand up alone from it (one and a half times length of leg from knee to foot, or 130° angle of the knee should accomplish this). Have patient place both of his hands on the table. Stand up unassisted for about ten seconds then sit for approximately fifteen seconds. Repeat ten times, increasing the number as the patient's endurance increases. Practice standing balance at the same time.
11. Quadriceps.
12. Sitting balance exercise.

When you are satisfied that you understand the information in this unit, please continue.

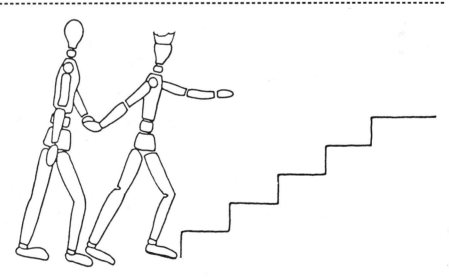

You and Mr. Jones have ONE more step to climb on the Independence Staircase of Progressive Mobilization. *The patient needs to learn to walk.*

Please turn to the next Section, Gait Training, or "How to Teach Your Patient to Walk."

Gait Training, or "How To Teach Your Patient to Walk"

Safety First: 5 Rules

Safety Rule 1: Are You Ready to Teach Your Patient to Walk? Is Your Patient Ready?

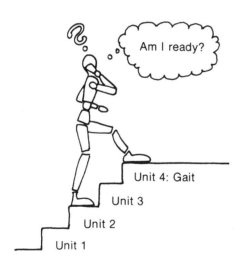

It is very important that you have prepared your patient well for walking. Preparation means that he is able to perform all the activities discussed in the other three sections of the Progressive Mobilization Chapter. It means that he has taken *every step* necessary on the Independence Staircase.

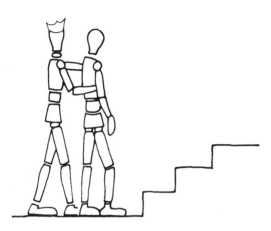

Could you get from the bottom to the top of a flight of stairs without climbing the steps in between? Of course not. To determine if Mr. Jones *is ready* to walk, ask *three important questions.*

Question: 1. Mr. Jones, *can you sit*? Show me.

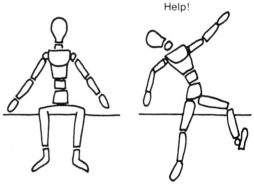

If your patient looks like the first picture, proceed. If he looks like the second, go back and teach him how to sit alone with good sitting balance.

Question: 2. Mr. Jones, *can you stand up*? Do you have good strong legs? Show me.

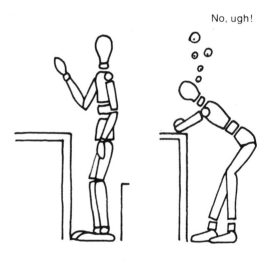

If your patient looks like the left picture, proceed. If he looks like the right one, go back and teach him how to stand and strengthen his legs.

Question: 3. Mr. Jones, *can you stand* and *balance* alone? Show me.

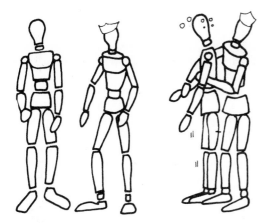

If your patient looks like the left picture, proceed. If he looks like the right one, go back and perfect his standing balance.

It is important that your patient *at least* be able to stand and balance himself before he tries to walk. It is best that strengthening, balance, and endurance building exercises be continued in conjunction with the walking program so the patient will develop as much strength as possible.

We are cautioning you to prepare your patient properly for walking because, *if you do not*, walking will prove to be taxing, unsafe, depressing, and, perhaps, futile.

You should use all the units of this Progressive Mobilization chapter properly. Be sure that your patient is ready for each step on the Independence Staircase. If you have prepared your patient well, walking or gait training can be a rewarding and fun experience for both of you. Can you recall a moment when you saw a child take his first step? Let your patient know you are proud of him. It really helps!

Safety Rule 2: SAFEST GAIT

In general, providing that the patient has been well prepared and given the proper walking aids, his instincts about walking will be correct as to safety and technique. As long as safety is not sacrificed, it is all right to experiment with modifications in his walking patterns. Where there is a choice between the speed or the appearance of gait and its safety, always choose the gait which is the safest.

Safety Rule 3: CARDIAC PRECAUTIONS

When you walk a patient you should monitor his pulse and watch for other cardiac signs during exercise. Do you remember the importance of this procedure? Review the first section of this chapter if you do not.

Safety Rule 4: GOOD SHOES

"A building is as good as its foundation." Your patient should be wearing *good shoes*. Shoes that slide off the patient's feet (scuffs, etc.), high heels, and slippery soles can lead to falls and sprained ankles. Your patient already has some kind of difficulty walking or he would not be here for your help, so do not add to his problems. See that he has good shoes. Tied oxfords with rubber heels are the best for men and women.

Safety Rule 5: CORRECT GUARDING

You are responsible for the patient's safety when he is walking. Described here is the safest and most appropriate way to *prevent falls* during walking. If you have prepared your patient well for walking by following Safety Rules 1 to 4 above, you will have eliminated most of the following hazards. But even then, you must anticipate them and be prepared to guard accordingly.

Most patients, particularly stroke victims, will fall toward their weak side if they are going to fall. Patients can also fall forward or backward. They fall primarily because their muscles are weak and their legs "crumble" under them or their balance is poor. Weakness in various muscles often makes it difficult to maintain the proper position for walking.

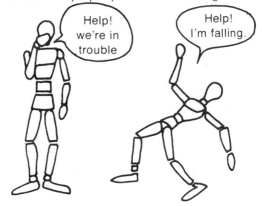

Following is a description of how you should look while guarding. In our example, Mr. Jones' left side is the weakest. *Stand on his left side* and *just a little behind him.* Put your right hand on his belt or walking belt and your left hand on the front of his shoulder. In this position you can push back on his shoulder and push forward on his hips to straighten him up, or pull him against yourself. If you cannot hold him, you are in a good position to *ease* him *gently* to the floor. Remember to use good body mechanics. If a patient is falling, you can do more harm to your back and the patient by straining to hold him up than if you ease him to the floor. Back injuries will not help anyone. You should never hold a patient only by the arm or let him hold onto you, because if he suddenly starts to fall, you will both fall over.

As your patient's walking ability improves, gradually release your hold on him by taking your hand from his shoulder, and then from his belt, until he is on his own. *However, always* stand in the same position to catch him if necessary. *Practice* using this position until it *feels comfortable.* This is very important. If you do not feel comfortable and balanced, it will be hard for you to help your patient effectively.

Take a partner, stand in the guarding position, and practice walking with him. Keep your feet spread apart for good balance and take a step each time your partner does: coordinate your steps with his. Practice until *you feel* comfortable.

When guarding a patient, be careful that you do not hold onto him so much that he does not have freedom of movement. Remember that you are there to teach and assist him to walk, not to drag him around the room!

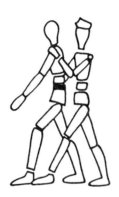

Test for Safety First: 5 Rules

Please answer the following questions regarding safety during gait before continuing.

1. *Name three activities that your patient should be able to do before he can walk.*
   a. _____
   b. _____
   c. _____
2. *Why should you prepare your patient well for walking?* _____

3. *If Mr. Jones' pulse is 122 while sitting in the wheelchair, is he safe to walk?* _____
4. *State what type of shoes are best for patients to wear.* _____

5. *Describe the guarding position for walking.* _____
   _____

6. *Can this section of the Progressive Mobilization package be used completely alone?* _____
   Why or why not? _____

If you answered as follows you were correct:

1. a. *Sit alone—good sitting balance.*
   b. *Stand up easily—good leg strength.*
   c. *Balance alone—good standing balance.*

2. *Otherwise he might fail and the effort for walking would be taxing, unsafe, depressing, and futile.*
3. *No, his cardiac status is not stable.*
4. *Tied oxfords with rubber heels.*
5. *Stand on patient's weak side, to the side and a little behind. Place one hand on belt, other hand on front of shoulder.*
6. *No, because he must be able to perform all the steps or activities on the Independence Staircase in order to succeed with gait.*

Normal Gait

Ideally our attempts at gait training are designed to teach our patients to walk as normally as possible. Often due to a patient's diagnosis, he is not able to perform these normal movements. For you to determine what normal is, a brief discussion of normal gait follows. Recall that this book is not intended to be a physical therapy text, and gait is discussed here only as it applies basically for our needs.

During normal gait, each leg alternates between *stance phase,* during which the leg is on the ground, and *swing phase*, during which the leg is brought from behind to the forward position. Each phase has distinct characteristics, many of which are very important to teach the patient so he will be able to walk effectively and efficiently. Each step is discussed in the order that it occurs during normal gait.

Stance Phase

1. *Heel Strike.* Normally we hit the floor with our heel first and with our foot dorsiflexed (left picture). Patients occasionally will attempt to touch with their toes first and are usually best encouraged to follow the normal pattern. This is especially important to consider during crutch walking. If the patients strike the floor with their toes first, normal action of the foot

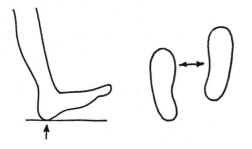

cannot follow; and their gait pattern becomes awkward, unstable, and inefficient. When the foot hits the floor, it should be pointed straight ahead, with the knee in full extension, and the leg slightly abducted (feet apart) (right picture).

2. *Stance.* After the heel strike, the patient rolls over onto the ball of his foot, and bends slightly (about 15°) at the knee. He then *fully extends the knee.* He must be able to stand

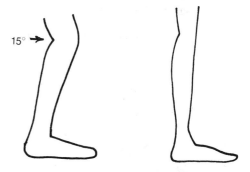

straight on that leg. A strong quadriceps muscle or an assistive device might be needed to produce this stance position for the patient to be able to walk. If the knee "buckles" at this point, the other leg cannot be lifted off the floor.

Also during stance, the trunk must be maintained in an upright position to move the other leg. This is accomplished by the action of the gluteus maximus muscle. If the gluteus maximus is not functioning when the involved leg is in stance position, the trunk falls forward. To compensate for this weakness the patient must be instructed to stand very straight with his shoulders back and his pelvis forward. You might need to assist your patient in maintaining this position initially. Review the guarding position. You will notice that you are standing in a perfect position to assist the patient with this problem. (See illustrations on next page.)

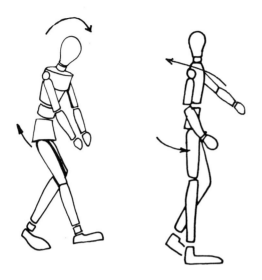

can be called "a functional long leg." This means simply that the patient for some reason cannot "shorten" the length of his leg by the normal movements discussed above to swing that leg past the other one. The leg will often feel "glued to the floor." Reasons for a functional long leg may be long leg casts or braces, stiff knee joints, weak ankles (drop foot), weak or nonfunctioning hip flexors, plantar flexion contractures, etc. What to do about the problem of a functional long leg will be discussed under Assistive Devices, pp. 87-88.

3. *Push Off:* The patient then pushes off with his toes and the ball of his foot, bends his knee slightly, and simultaneously bends his hip slightly.

This action proceeds into the *swing phase.*

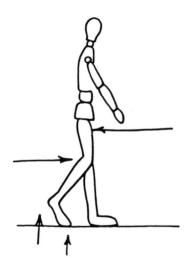

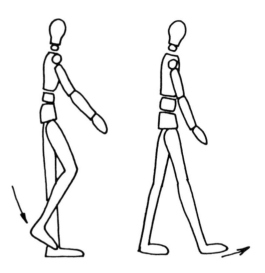

Swing Phase

The other leg is now in stance phase.

1. With the hip and knee bent, the ankle and foot held at about a 90° angle, and the body weight shifted onto the other leg, the leg begins to swing forward.

    If a patient cannot perform one, two, or more of these normal movements, the leg

2. When the leg swings past the other leg, the knee extends by a combined action of the hamstrings to control the speed of the extension, and the quadriceps muscle to produce full extension of the knee. All steps produced are equal in length. (If the quadriceps and hamstrings do not function properly here, the patient will not produce full extension of the knee and not swing the leg completely past the other leg; and/or when heel strike occurs the knee will "pop" back into forced hyperextension.)

3. With the knee straight, the foot dorsiflexes beyond a 90° angle, and the patient's leg is again in a position for heel strike. The gait pattern repeats.

As one can imagine, all patients will present a different problem with their gait pattern. One patient might be able to dorsiflex his foot for heel strike and to clear his foot during swing phase but not be able to flex his hip; another might be able to do both but not extend his knee. It is our responsibility to help the patient become as normal as possible and to find ways that the patient can walk regardless of his inability to follow the normal gait pattern precisely. We might need to strengthen a particular muscle or muscle group to correct the gait problem, or substitute an assistive device for the inability to perform a certain movement, or instruct the patient to use walkers, crutches, or canes. Whatever we decide to do to help the patient, *remember two points*.

1. we want the patient to become as normal as possible within the limits of his diagnosis, and
2. we must produce a gait that is as *safe* and *functional* as possible.

Continue reading now about assistive devices and how to use walking aids to help the patient become as normal and functional as possible. Recall previous units, which discuss ways of strengthening muscle groups to achieve this effect.

Assistive Devices

Lifts

A *lift* can be placed on the patient's good or uninvolved leg. This *makes* the uninvolved leg longer than the involved leg and, in theory, "equalizes" the "functional" longer length of the involved leg. The patient can then swing the involved leg past the uninvolved one and produce a more normal gait.

Lifts can be made from any rigid material by tracing the patient's shoe shape, cutting it out, and taping it to the bottom of the patient's shoe with masking tape. The height of the lift depends on how much length needs to be added to the good leg in order to allow the other leg to swing through. Start with a quarter-inch lift and add height until the patient can move his leg. Try not to exceed three quarters of an inch because this could disturb his balance. On the other hand, do not be afraid to add more if it is absolutely necessary, especially with a long leg cast or a stiff knee. As the patient's gait improves, try to decrease the height of the lift. You may be able to abandon it later as the patient learns to move his leg. If it is obvious that the patient should always have some type of lift, a shoe repair shop can add the height he needs.

Can you see how this would help your young patient with a long leg cast to use crutches, or your stroke patient to use his cane? Or a patient with a weak hip flexor and hip musculature move his leg forward?

Braces

Have you ever seen a patient (most likely a stroke patient) who dragged his toe when walking? This problem is called a "dropped foot." It is usually due to muscle weakness or lack of muscle function in the ankle. The patient cannot move his ankle up and down or from side to side. Dropped foot causes great instability in the foot and a functional long leg. These problems can make gait difficult or impossible. A short leg brace provides an easy remedy. It stabilizes the ankle at the 90° angle and holds it from moving improperly from side to side. The patient can then move his leg properly and without fear of a twisted ankle.

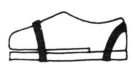

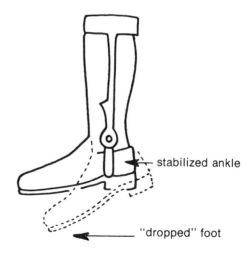

— stabilized ankle

"dropped" foot

A brace is not necessarily a substitute for a lift, nor is a lift a substitute for a brace. One or the other or both could be needed for your patient. Experiment and decide. Let the patient have some input into the decision as well. Remember, the patient's instincts concerning safety of gait are generally good.

Knee Immobilizers

If the patient cannot keep his knee sufficiently extended during stance phase to allow proper swing phase on the other side, a knee immobilizer will enable him to do so. A knee immobilizer can be purchased from your local medical supply vendor. For it to be effective in keeping the leg straight, the knee immobilizer must have heavy stays and a strap across the patella.

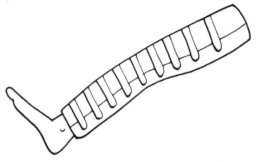

The knee immobilizer is a temporary device and used as such permits early gait training and stimulus to the quadriceps muscle. If the ankle dorsiflexors are weak or absent as well, the knee immobilizer can be used along with a short leg brace.

At intervals, attempts should be made to remove the knee immobilizer as the patient's leg becomes stronger. When the knee remains sufficiently straight during stance phase, the knee immobilizer can be removed completely. If it is apparent that the patient will not be able to keep his knee extended sufficiently during stance phase, a long leg brace with a knee lock could be needed.

Notice that the use of a knee immobilizer or a long leg brace with a locked knee will produce the "functional long leg" discussed, and a lift on the good foot should be used to help compensate for it.

Remember these points! We have had patients come to the rehabilitation center because they could not walk. All we did was to provide them with a lift or a brace and their walking problem was solved. Do you see the value of knowing what the patient needs?

Walking Aids

Crutches, Walkers, Canes, or You.

How do we know whether a patient needs a walking aid and, if so, what kind? The following table can be used as a quick reference for determining your patient's needs. Study it carefully. When using any walking aid, the patient should:

1. lean hard on it to get the full benefit of the device;
2. lean on it less as he progresses in ability (except, of course, with crutches or walkers for nonweight-bearing fractures); and
3. move it with the weak leg.

TABLE 2-3
Walking Aids

TYPE	DESCRIPTION	WHICH PATIENTS SHOULD USE THEM	COMMENTS
Walker			
a. Standard Walker	Rubber tips Can be adjusted to proper height	Patients with general weakness Patients with two good arms The older patient Patients with general mild balance problems Patients with a fractured hip, leg or foot Patients with weak legs or leg	The walker must be lifted when moved. It is very stable.

TABLE 2-3 (Continued)

TYPE	DESCRIPTION	WHICH PATIENTS SHOULD USE THEM	COMMENTS
b. Gliding Walker 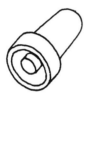	Same as on previous page except it has metal plates on tips instead of rubber	All above plus Patient with poor forward and backward balance Parkinsonism Arthritis	The walker may be pushed or slid on floor The patient with poor forward and backward balance does not have to lift this walker. When he does have to lift a walker, he tends to fall backward
Crutches			
a. Crutches 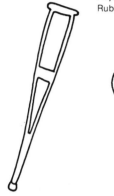	Wooden or steel Adjustable Rubber tips	Younger patient Fractured hip, feet, etc. Needs *two strong arms* Needs *good balance*	Not recommended for older patients Crutches are *only* as stable as the person using them
Canes			
a. Walkcane 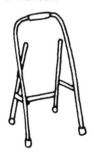	4 legs Rubber tips Adjustable	Hemiplegic patient Patient with only *one* good arm Patient who has a lot of lateral instability (keeps falling to one side—hemiplegic patient primarily) Patient who needs to take weight off of an involved foot, e.g., sprained ankle, weakness Patient with general balance problems	This cane provides much more stability than a regular cane Recommend it as the first device used in progress toward independence without a cane Use in hand opposite the involved leg When used strictly for balance problems, use it in the hand which is most effective for the patient. Let him try it and see!
b. walkcane with glider tips 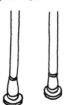	Same as above except has glider tips	All the above	Even better with balance problems, it can be pushed (see walker with gliders)

TABLE 2-3 (Continued)

TYPE	DESCRIPTION	WHICH PATIENTS SHOULD USE THEM	COMMENTS
c. Quad cane		Patients with same problems as listed under walkcanes but less severe	Gives less support than a walkcane does Used as the second device in progress toward independence without a cane
d. Cane		Patients same as above but even *less severe*	Pictured here is the best type of cane. It is the most stable of all regular canes. Gives less support than a quad cane Use as a third device to independence
You a. Guarding	You are in the position described in Safety Rule No. 5 or, just allow the patient to hold your hand	Patient with very mild balance problems Confused patient Patient who just progressed from a cane Patient who needs a little support for confidence	Sometimes these people need to use a cane They cannot understand what to do with a walker They may fall over a walker and this is unsafe
b. Standby	Walk in guarding position but do not touch patient	Patient is doing better than above	Almost to independence
c. Let him walk alone		Patient is doing better still	Independence!

You have been given a lot of information that is basic to gait training. Refer back to it as you continue to learn the techniques of teaching a patient to walk. Here are some questions to review your understanding of this material.

1. *What patient would need a lift?* _____
_____

2. *In normal gait, do you land on your heel first, or your toes first?* _____
_____

3. *Your patient has poor forward and backward balance. Which walking aid would you use?* _____

4. *You should move the walking aid with the* _____ *leg.*

5. *Which cane would you use for a patient who needed a lot of support laterally?* ___
_____
_____

6. *Where would you stand to guard a patient?*
_____

7. *Should you change a patient's gait pattern that is safe but does not look normal?* ___ *Why or why not?* _____

8. *What causes a "functional long leg?"* ___
_____
_____

Answers:

1. *A person with a functional long leg.*
2. *Heel first.*
3. *Walker—preferably glider walker.*
4. *Weak.*
5. *Walkcane.*
6. *Weak side, and a little behind him.*
7. *No, you should never sacrifice safety for appearance.*
8. *Weak leg muscles, stiff joints, tight muscles, long leg braces.*

If you answered correctly, you are doing well. Use this information as we continue. If you made some errors, review the material before you proceed.

The nurse is setting the scene for "how to stand a patient from a chair," but before we continue, look at the way we have divided the remaining instruction:

1. How to stand a patient from a chair.
2. How to measure a patient for a walking aid.
3. How to use a walking aid.
4. How to turn around using a walking aid.
5. How to back up, and how to sit down in a chair.

We're at the top of the independence staircase and we're anxious to learn this step!

Walking

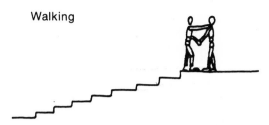

How to Stand a Patient from a Chair

Set the scene.

1. Mr. Jones' shoes are on. He is wearing good ones.
2. His chair is stabilized with wheelchair brakes locked (for greater stability, push chair against a wall also).
3. All stools or foot plates are out of the way so he will not trip or hit his legs against anything.
4. His pulse is taken; cardiac signs are good.
5. His walking aid (walker, crutches, or cane) is in its appropriate position (to be discussed later).

The nurse:

1. "Mr. Jones, slide forward in your chair and put your feet flat on the floor" (first picture). *Note:* If the patient cannot slide forward in the chair, instruct him to stretch out his legs in front of him, lean back against the chair and push his back against it. This will allow his hips to slide forward (middle picture). Then he can pull his body forward by grasping on the chair arm or seat (right picture).

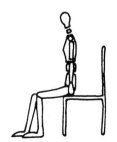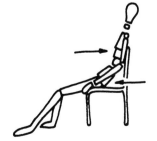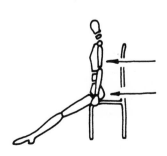

2. "Now put both hands on the arms of the chair, or, put one hand on the walker or crutches, and one hand on the chair."
3. "Lean forward a little, *push* with your arms, straighten your legs and back, and stand up straight."

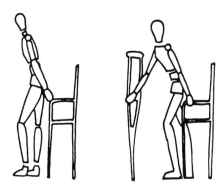

4. "Now put both hands on the walking aid (if appropriate)—either one at a time or both at once."

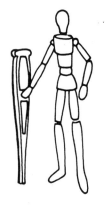
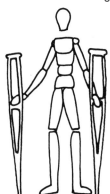
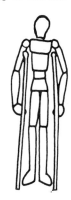

5. "Get your balance. You are ready for the next step."

Note: On occasion, you may need to vary this method of getting a patient out of the chair. For example:

1. If he has a long leg cast or hip fracture, he cannot put both his legs under him.
2. If the patient has only one arm, he can only push with the one arm. Be sure it is on the chair.

Two variations using walking aids are:

1. *To stand up with a regular cane.* Hold the cane in one hand while using both hands on the chair.
2. *To stand up with crutches.* Hold both crutches in one hand by the handgrips. Put the other hand on the arm of the chair and follow the original procedure. When you are standing, take one crutch and put it under the opposite arm. Then turn the other crutch into position. The patient should be standing as shown.

Test for How to Stand a Patient From a Chair

Here are a few questions to see if you have understood the directions for standing up.

1. *Where do you tell Mr. Jones to push?* ____
   _____
2. *How should he position his legs?* _____
   _____
   _____
3. *What is important to remember about the wheelchair when a patient stands?* _____
   _____
   _____

If you answered:

1. *on the arms of the wheelchair,*
2. *under him—knees bent to at least 90°,*
3. *brakes locked and stabilized,*

you were correct. Review anything you did not understand.

Good. Now you have your patient standing. How does the walking aid look? Is it all right? Too tall? Too short? How to answer these questions will be discussed in the next section.

How to Measure Walking Aids

The proper measurement of a walking aid is important if the patient is to walk properly. Here are five rules that apply to measuring equipment.

1. *Measurements Should be Taken Standing.* You can estimate the measurements of walking aids before the patient stands, but the final measurement must come when the patient is standing. That is why we discussed standing first!
2. *Trust the Patient's Instincts.* You do want the walking aid to fit the patient correctly "by the book", but how the patient feels is equally important. If the fit is close to what is theoretically correct and the patient is holding the device properly, let the patient try it his way.
3. *Be Sure Legs Are Even.* Adjustable walkers and canes can be adjusted by pushing in on the button and sliding the tubing in or out to make the walker or cane shorter or longer, respectively. A "wobbly" walking aid is worse than none. Adjustable crutches have screws and wing nuts, which are pulled out to move the handgrips or lengthen the crutches. Be sure that these are replaced tightly. Do not leave any space showing between the different pieces of the crutches, or the screws could break.
4. *Be Sure Parts Are Clean.* Always check the rubber tips on walkers, crutches, and canes. They should be clean and not worn. They should have suction ability and lots of tread: worn rubber tips can cause slipping accidents.
5. *Be Sure Patients Have Shoes.* Always measure the patient with shoes on and, preferably, with the shoes that he will wear for walking.

Keep these rules in mind while you learn how to measure walking aids.

Walkers

1. Place walker in front of patient and partially around him.
2. He should stand straight, shoulders relaxed.
3. His elbows should be *almost straight.*

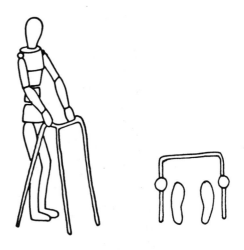

4. Let him try the walker. See if he can push on it easily without bending over.
5. Keep readjusting the walker until it feels right and he can use it well.

Note: Often, people measure walkers too high and the patients get very tired trying to lift their weight with their arms.

Practice: If a walker is available try one that is too high for you. Then try one which is too low, and finally one that fits. Do you not agree that the walker is harder to use when it is too high or too low?

Crutches

1. Have the patient hold the crutches with the tips about six inches from each foot and out to the side in a good comfortable weight-bearing position.

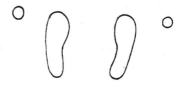

2. He should stand straight, shoulders relaxed.
3. The axillary pads should lie against the ribs about three to four finger widths from the axilla or armpits.
4. The handles should be positioned so the elbows are about 160° extended, or about even with the greater trochanter.

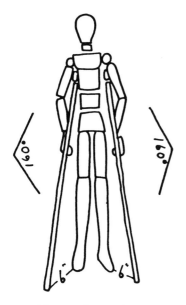

weight should go onto the hands! *Not* the armpits!

Canes

1. Patient should stand straight, shoulders relaxed, with one hand on the cane.
2. Hold the cane in a good weight-bearing position (approximately five to six inches ahead and to the side of the patient's foot).

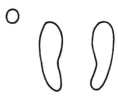

Again consider comfort and use.

Note: NEVER let the patient press down on the axillary pads. Weight bearing on the axillary pads could paralyze his arms from pressure on the nerves that run in the axilla. All

3. The hand holding the top of the cane should rest so the elbows are about 160° extended, or about even with the greater trochanter.
4. Consider the patient's feelings about his ability to push on the cane.

Test for How to Measure Walking Aids

Do you think that you could measure a patient for a walking aid now? See the questions below to be sure.

1. *How far from the armpits should the top of the crutches be?* _____
   Why? _____
   _____

2. *What position should the elbows be in for crutches, canes, walkers?* _____
   _____
   _____

3. *What should be your final criteria for walking aids?* _____
   _____
   _____

4. *Briefly describe how the rubber tips on a walking aid should look.* _____
   _____
   _____

5. *Walking aids should be measured when the patient is* _____
   and wearing _____.

Check here to see how you did on the questions.

1. *Three to four finger widths, so the patient does not lean on crutch tops with his armpits.*
2. *About 160° extended or even with the greater trochanter.*
3. *That the patient feels comfortable and he can use the walking aid easily.*
4. *Not worn, good suction, clean, lots of tread.*
5. *Standing, shoes.*

Now that Mr. Jones is standing and measured with his walking aid, we are going to watch him and the nurse walk down the hall.

Using Walking Aids

Walking with a Walker

The nurse:

Are you ready Mr. Jones? Now remember you have broken your right leg and cannot put any weight on it. However, you can place your foot on the floor while you walk. We are going to use a standard walker.

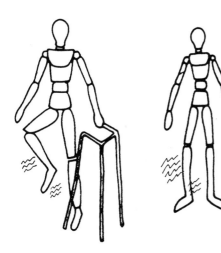

You stood up very well, Mr. Jones. Do you feel balanced? Practicing those stand-ups and standing balance exercises has helped. You are getting very strong.

Stand straight and look straight ahead. Pick the walker up, and place it forward a little. Put your right foot forward, and place it on the floor. No weight, please. Push *hard* on your hands; and, lifting all of your weight, step forward with your left foot, placing it next to the right foot. Repeat these same actions for each step.

1. Move walker forward

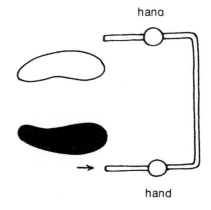

hand

hand

2. Move right foot (involved foot)

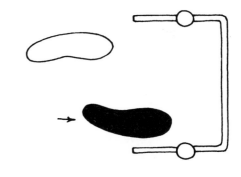

3. Move left foot (uninvolved foot)

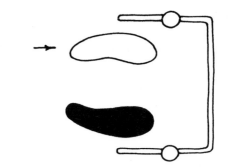

Repeat

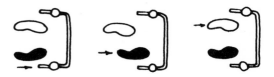

Note:

1. Remember your guarding position and body mechanics.
2. Be sure the walker is always ahead of the patient. Do not let him step up against the front bar of the walker because this is an unstable position for the walker.
3. If the patient has poor forward-backward balance, use a walker with gliders so he does not have to pick the walker up off the floor.
4. If the patient has a weak leg or a partial weight-bearing fracture, use the same method described with this exception: that the patient puts some weight on his leg as well as his hands. As the weak leg becomes stronger, he gradually increases the weight on his leg and decreases the weight supported by his hands. For a fractured leg, this progression should be guided by a physician.
5. Some patients will have to hold their leg off the floor. If they are confused and touch their foot to the floor, even lightly, they may end up with all their weight on that leg. Sometimes a *lift* on the *uninvolved leg* is helpful because this will make the involved leg much shorter and they will remember not to step on it, plus the lift will make it easier to move the fractured leg.

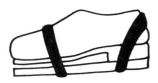

Answer the following questions.

1. *Should you let a patient step up to the front bar of the walker?* _____

   _____

   Why or why not? _____

   _____

2. *Name the sequence of the movements carried out with the walker.* _____
   _____ *then,*
   _____ *then,*
   _____ *then,*
   _____ *then, repeat.*

3. *The patient must* _____ *with his arms.*

Answers:

1. *No—because the walker is unstable in that position.*
2. *Move walker, move involved leg, push on the walker, move uninvolved leg.*
3. *Push hard.*

Walking with Crutches

The nurse:

> Balance with crutches is very important, Mr. Jones. Press on the crutch handles so you become accustomed to pushing on them. Remember, when you walk, do not push on the crutches under your armpits.
>
> Mr. Jones, you have a cast on your right leg so you cannot put your foot on the floor. Hold it up off the floor.
>
> Do you see the triangle that your crutches are making with your feet?

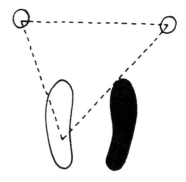

The triangular position of feet and crutches make you stable on them. *Never* line the crutches up with your feet. This position is like walking on a tight-rope.

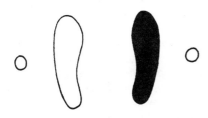

Always keep your triangle either forward or backward.

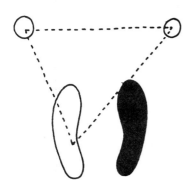

Forward

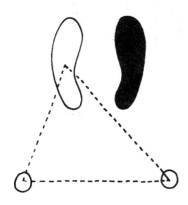

Backward

When you are walking, Mr. Jones, hold up your right foot, put both crutches forward, push on your hands, and step past the crutches with your left foot landing on your heel first (heel strike) for balance.

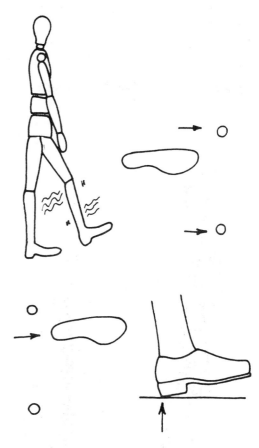

See the backward triangle now? Repeat these steps again. Use momentum from one step to the next to make the crutch walking easier. In other words, repeat one step immediately after the other. If you stop after each step, walking with crutches will be very hard work!

If Mr. Jones could put weight on his involved foot, you would tell him to (1) move his crutches forward; (2) step forward with his involved foot up to the crutches, then; (3) step past the crutches with his uninvolved foot, landing on his heel first.

Start:

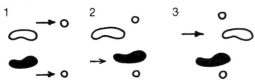

As he becomes stronger he will move the crutches and the involved foot all at once (three-point crutch gait).

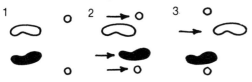

If the patient cannot step past the crutches, he might use them like a walker. He would only step up to them and not past them. If this were the case, I would recommend that your patient use a walker instead of crutches. Remember: Do not line up *both* crutches and *both* feet.

All these examples are designed to be used with patients who have a weak, or a non-weight-bearing leg. There are other variations of crutch gaits that can be used as your patient's legs become stronger or as he is able to bear considerable weight on his leg. These gait patterns resemble cane walking and are shown below. Follow the arrows to determine when to move each foot (Figures 2-9 to 2-11).

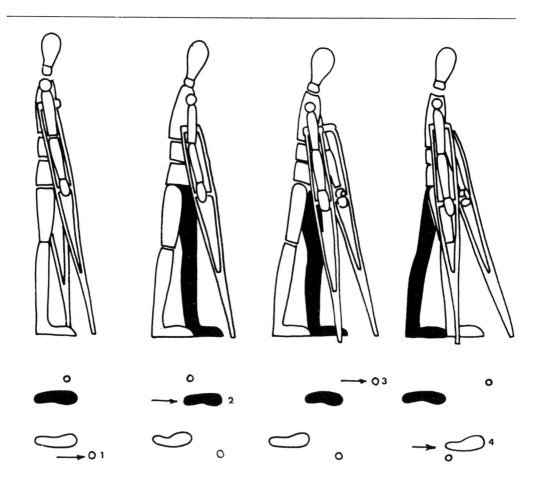

Figure 2-9 Moving one crutch, or one foot, at a time.

Four-point crutch gait (opposite crutch first pattern). This crutch gait is very stable.

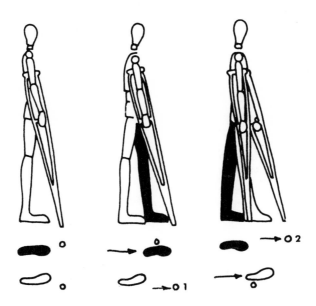

Figure 2-10 **Moving one crutch and one foot together.**

Two-point crutch gait (crutch and opposite foot together pattern). This gait is faster than moving one crutch and then one foot separately, as in the four-point crutch gait.

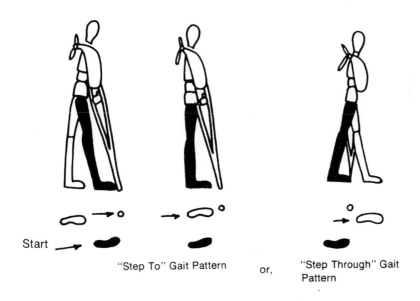

Start

"Step To" Gait Pattern   or,   "Step Through" Gait Pattern

Figure 2-11 **Using only one crutch and moving one crutch and one foot together.**

(See cane section for how to do this.)

Answer these three questions to see how you are doing.

1. *Name two important facts to remind patients regarding walking with crutches.*

   a. _____
   _____

   b. _____
   _____

2. *When you take the step with your uninvolved foot you should land on your _____ first. Why?_____*
   _____

3. *Move the crutches with the _____ _____ leg.*

Answers:

1. a. *Never put weight on crutch tops—this puts pressure on nerves in armpits.*
   b. *Do not line up both crutches and both feet.*
2. *Heel, balance is better.*
3. *Involved, or bad.*

Did you get them all correct? Continue when you are ready.

Walking with Canes

Cane gait is very similar to crutch gait and is further along in the progression toward independence. The three types of canes discussed here (walkcane, quad canes, and regular canes) are also used progressively.

If a patient needs a great deal of support you would start with the walkcane because it has four, standardlike legs. As the patient becomes stronger he can progress to a quad cane (which gives less support) and then to a regular cane.

As with crutches, there should always be a triangle with the cane and the feet. In addition, the cane should *always* be used in the hand opposite the weak leg.

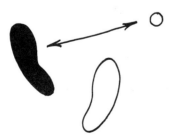

Canes give patients lateral support. A good example is the patient with a left hemiplegia. He would tend to fall to the left. Good use of the cane in the right hand would encourage him to lean to the right, making him more stable laterally.

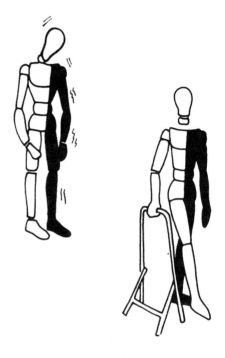

If Mr. Jones has had a stroke and needed to use a walkcane, these would be his instructions from the nurse. (Remember good body mechanics and the guarding position.)
The nurse:

> Mr. Jones, move the cane forward and out to the side. Put your weight on it, shifting the weight off the involved leg. Move your involved leg up even with the cane. Be sure that your feet are spread apart. Then, press on the cane and, putting as much weight as possible on your involved leg, step past the cane with your uninvolved leg.

This could be called *cane first gait* (step-through gait pattern).

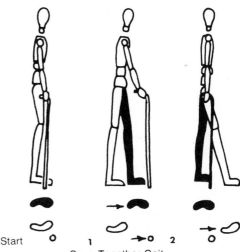

Start   o   1   →

Cane First Gait

Start   o   1   → o   2   → o

Cane Together Gait

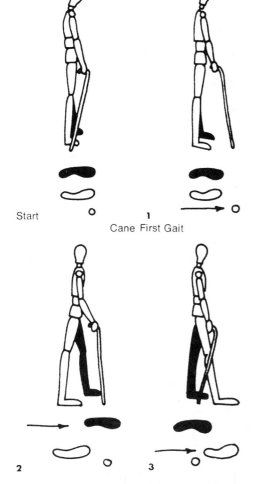

2   o   3   o

If your patient's balance or strength is not good enough to step past the walkcane or cane, teach him a *step-to gait*. But be sure to keep the walkcane well ahead of the feet.

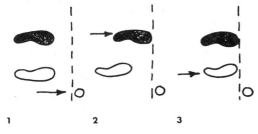

1   2   3

The stronger, well-coordinated patient should move the cane and his involved foot forward at the same time and then step past the cane with his uninvolved foot. This could be called the *cane together gait*.

Remember, when using any of these walking aids, try to have the patient walk as normally as possible without sacrificing safety (Safety Rule 2, p. 83). At first, your patient will not be able to walk very far; but as he practices, his endurance will increase, and he will be able to walk further. Encourage your patient to walk a little further every day!

Here are some review questions:

1. *Which cane gives the most stability?*

_____

2. *Your patient has a left hemiplegia. In which hand should he hold the cane?*

_____

3. *Repeat the sequence used for cane gait.*
   a. _____

   b. _____

   c. _____

4. *Canes give stability in which direction?* __

_____

Check your answers.

Answers:
1. *Walkcane.*
2. *Right hand.*
3. a. *Move cane forward and out to the side.*
   b. *Step forward with involved foot—even with the cane.*
   c. *Step past the cane with the uninvolved foot.*
4. *Laterally.*

How to Turn Around Using Walking Aids

The method of turning around is the same regardless of which walking aid Mr. Jones uses. In this instance, Mr. Jones is using a walker.

The nurse:

> Mr. Jones, always turn toward your good side. Move the walker around in a small circle, using the same gait pattern as for straight walking. (Keep the uninvolved foot in the inside of the circle.) First move your walker and turn it a little. Then, step with your involved foot, now move your uninvolved foot. Repeat until you are turned around.

How to Back Up and How to Sit Down in a Chair

Set the scene:

1. wheelchair locked, or regular chair stabilized;
2. foot plates up, out of the way;
3. Mr. Jones will use a walker in this episode.

The nurse:

> Walk up close to the chair (bed, toilet, etc.) and turn around again. Be sure that the foot plates of your wheelchair are out of the way and that the wheelchair is locked. Turn around until *your back is toward the chair.* Now, *back up with your walker.* Move your walker backwards toward you. Press on your hands. Step back with your good foot, then move your bad foot back. Repeat these steps until you feel the *back of both of your legs* against the seat of the chair. (See illustrations on next page.)

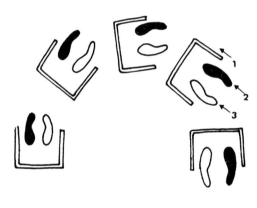

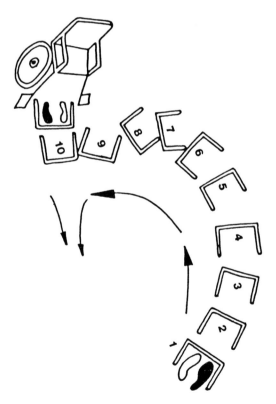

For safety, do not pivot on the good or uninvolved foot—walk in a circle as shown above. Be sure to keep the feet spread apart when turning. If the feet get too close together, the patient is likely to lose his balance and fall over.

"Good, Mr. Jones. That was a nice turn. Head back to your chair and I will teach you . . . ."

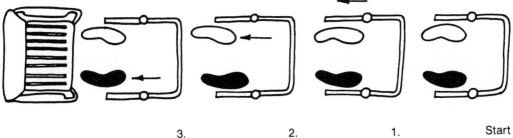

3.   2.   1.   Start

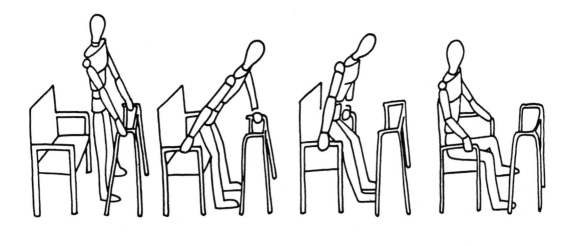

1.   2.   3.   4.

Be sure that the chair is stable. Are the brakes locked? Let go of the walker with one hand, and reach back to the arm of the chair. Holding firmly to the wheelchair with that hand, reach back with the other hand. Using both your arms and legs, lean forward a little and ease yourself down into the chair. Slide back in the chair until you are in a comfortable position.

There you are safe and sound, Mr. Jones! Let me check your pulse. It is good.

Described above is the correct way to turn around, and sit down in a chair using a walking aid. No deviations from this method should be allowed when a patient is using crutches or a walker. Turning around is probably the most hazardous time whenever a patient is walking. If they do not perform the turning process carefully, their feet get too close together, they lose their balance and fall. Many broken hips have occurred when a patient has turned to sit down into a chair.

Sitting Down with Crutches

If Mr. Jones had been using crutches, to sit down he would first take the crutches from under his arms and put them both in one hand. Then, holding onto the handgrips, he could reach back with the other hand to the chair and continue as described above. This method is the reverse of standing up with crutches.

Turning to Sit When Not Using Walking Aids

If the patient is not using any walking aid or is using a quad cane or a regular cane, a second method of turning around to sit down in a chair is appropriate. In this instance, our patient has paralysis of his arm and leg on the left.

1. The patient walks up close to the chair facing it.
2. He places his cane to the side, being certain he has placed it so it will not fall in his way.
3. He holds onto the left arm of the chair with his uninvolved right hand.
4. He assures himself that his balance is good.
5. He then reaches across with his right hand grasping the right arm of the chair. He turns his feet carefully in a small circle, first moving his right foot, then his left, being certain that his feet are spread apart. His "good" or uninvolved side is always closest to the chair.
6. He continues to turn until he feels the chair touching the back of *both* of his legs and then he proceeds to sit down.

Our Mr. Jones has completed the entire walking process from getting up properly, to walking properly, to sitting down properly. He has really made it to the top of the Independence Staircase!

You and Mr. Jones have really done well. Let's see how you do with these questions.

1. Which direction should a patient turn if he is using a walking aid? _____
_____

2. Name two ways that a patient should move his feet when using a walking aid to turn or back up.
   a. _____
   b. _____

3. List the sequence of steps for a patient to use when sitting down in a chair.
   a. _____
   b. _____
   _____
   c. _____
   _____
   d. _____

4. When sitting down what precaution should be taken with the wheelchair?
_____

Your answers should be:

1. Toward his strongest or good side.
2. a. Same pattern as straight gait.
   b. Feet spread apart.
3. a. Turn around.
   b. Back up until he feels the back of the chair against the back of his legs.
   c. Reach back with one hand, then the other.
   d. Lean forward and sit down.
4. The brakes should be locked.

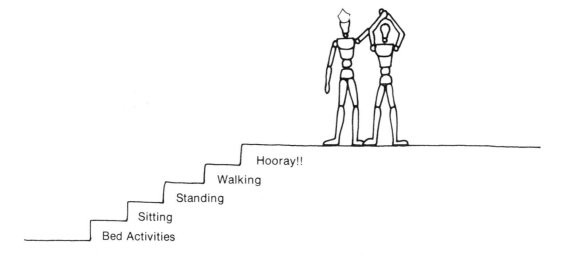

Hooray!!
Walking
Standing
Sitting
Bed Activities

Did you do well? Do you understand now how to walk a patient? If you have answered the questions along the way, I'm sure you do. Before we close, here are a few last-minute notes about walking.

At first the patient may only be able to walk a short distance and not have the strength or energy to turn or back up at all. In that case you should simply walk him forward as far as he can and then bring a chair up behind him to sit in. But *always*, no matter what type of patient, have him use the proper standing and sitting procedure.

Patients with poor lateral balance (usually stroke patients) have difficulty understanding the concept of leaning to the good side. This problem is most evident when a patient is using a cane but also occurs when they are using other walking aids also. Here is the solution:

Use two people. One does the instructing, encouraging the patient to lean on the cane or lean to the good side. The trick to getting the patient to do this is to hold him by the belt or under the arm and pull him toward you, forcing him to lean on his good side. The other person should stand in the guarding position but *not touch* the patient or talk to him. *All* the emphasis should be on the good side.

For patients with weak legs, assistive devices should be used progressively in the following order (imagine that the patient's legs are gradually getting stronger with exercise):

1. use a walker or crutches,
2. use a walkcane (start here for a stroke patient),
3. use a quad cane,
4. use a cane,
5. receive stand-by assistance from you,
6. independence.

Some patients might not make it beyond steps 1 or 2 of the progression. But, if they are doing their best and it is appropriate for their diagnosis, they have certainly succeeded (and so have you in teaching them).

Didn't it make you feel good to see the nurse and Mr. Jones in our book make it to the top of the Independence Staircase? You and your Mr. Jones can get there too! We have given you the information you need!

The Nurse and
  Mr. Jones

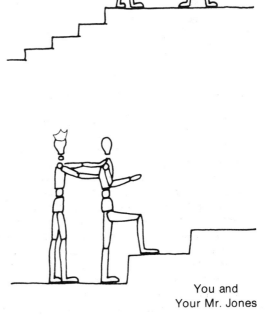

You and
Your Mr. Jones

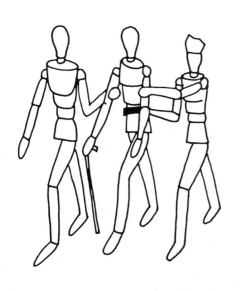

Posttest and Summary for Progressive Mobilization

Now that you have finished all sections of the Progressive Mobilization chapter, we would like to summarize the experience by giving you a few case histories to test your ability to develop a treatment plan. Remember to use the Independence Staircase and write down all the procedures you could follow with each patient to reach his particular goal. This will show you that you can help your Mr. Jones to independence. If you have trouble with this exercise, remember that the material is right here to review.

1. *Mrs. Brown is a 67-year old female with a fractured right hip. She had it pinned ten days ago. Her physician, Dr. Allen, tells you that he wants her to walk. What would you do?*_____

_____
_____
_____
_____
_____
_____
_____
_____
_____
_____
_____
_____
_____

2. *Today is May 3rd. Mr. Beech had a stroke on May 1st. Mr. Beech is alert, cooperative, has normal strength on the right, and fair strength on the left. His vital signs are normal. Dr. Anderson prescribes Progressive Mobilization activities. What would you do?* _____

_____
_____
_____
_____
_____
_____
_____
_____
_____
_____
_____
_____

Your answers to "What should you do" should be similar to these:

1. *Tell Mrs. Brown that you are going to help her walk. Take her pulse. Evaluate her arm strength. Evaluate her leg strength on the good side. See if Mrs. Brown can move her own involved leg. Check if she can move in bed alone, move sideways, sit up. Teach her anything with which she needs help. Be sure she has good shoes. Check sitting balance. Teach her how to transfer into the wheelchair without putting weight on her right leg. Check her standing ability. If it is good, proceed directly to using a walker. If not, do stand-ups and practice standing balance. (Could use crutches also, but at this age a walker is better.) Teach her to walk with the walker without putting weight on her right leg.*

2. *Tell Mr. Beech that you are going to begin activities with him that will allow him to regain his strength. Check his pulse. Check his range of motion, especially on his involved side. Do range of motion exercises as appropriate. Do active exercises to the left with emphasis on the ankle. Check his pulse after each activity and, if stable, continue. Ask him if he is tired. If not, continue. Check out his movements in bed and sitting balance. Be sure he has shoes. Check him for transfer ability and teach, if necessary. Transfer toward the right side. Check out his*

stand-up ability. Teach him stand-ups. Give him a walkcane on the right side. If he can walk with it easily (cane with opposite leg) try him with a regular cane, or none. As long as you keep checking pulse and other cardiac signs you can progress this patient very quickly.

Did your answers match? If they did not, please review the questions and answers again and keep in mind the Independence Staircase.

This is the end of your formal study in this area. You will find that as you use this method you will continue to learn. Each patient is different and each session with your patient will be a learning experience.

May we challenge you now to use the methods of treatment you have learned here? It is very rewarding to teach your patient, to be able to let go of his hand, and to see him walk independently. The nurse helped Mr. Jones to independence. Go ahead and help *your Mr. Jones* to independence too.

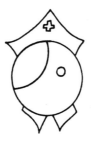

Techniques to
Facilitate
Communication

Joanna B. Chase, M.A.

3.

Introduction and Objectives

The overall goal of this chapter is to provide basic techniques to improve the flow of information between nurses and patients. It is not intended as an explanation of the causes, diagnosis, or treatment of speech disorders. If at all possible, patients with speech disorders should be referred to a qualified speech pathologist who holds a Certificate of Clinical Competence from the American Speech and Hearing Association. A list of qualified speech pathologists in your area can be obtained from the American Speech and Hearing Association, 9030 Old Georgetown Road, Washington, D.C. 20014.

After you have completed this chapter, you should be able to do the following:

1. Apply your knowledge of communication impairments and the ten techniques for facilitating communication in a testing situation.
2. Apply your knowledge of communication impairments and the ten techniques for facilitating communication in direct interaction with patients.

Communication Impairments

The communication process requires the ability to send and receive messages. The primary ways used to send information (output or expression) are speaking, gestures, and writing. Messages are received (input) by understanding the spoken word, interpreting gestures, and reading. Intact auditory, visual, and motor systems are necessary for the normal performance of these acts. An impairment in one or more of these systems will influence performance. The kind of impairment will determine the most effective kind of communication to use. A few of the more frequently encountered impairments will be briefly discussed.

Hearing (Input) Impairments

The hard of hearing patient utilizes visual cues to receive messages. Many of these patients are adept at speech reading and will respond appropriately when they are able to see the face of the speaker. Therefore, you should always stand directly in front of your patient when you are trying to communicate with him. This is particularly true with elderly patients, many of whom have a hearing loss called presbycusis. This type of loss is due to the aging process. It affects the higher sound frequencies and reduces the ability to discriminate speech. This is the "I hear you but I can't understand what you're saying" type of hearing problem, and increasing the loudness level does not improve reception. Patients who wear hearing aids should be encouraged to wear them while hospitalized and helped to put them on when needed. For the patient still unable to respond with the help of speech reading and gestures, written messages can be used.

Speech (Output) Impairments

Dysarthria

Damage to the central or peripheral nervous system that results in an impairment of the muscles controlling the speech structures causes a reduction in the intelligibility of speech. This reduction can range from speech that is only slightly slurred to speech that is totally unintelligible. Since the same structures are used for eating and speech, patients with dysarthria frequently have problems with chewing and swallowing. Encourage these patients to speak slowly and distinctly. If speech is still unintelligible, gestures or written responses can be used. For patients who cannot write because of motor impairments of arm and hand, a communication book using pictures of items needed for daily activities or an alphabet card for spelling words by pointing to the letters can be used.

Following a stroke, it is frequently found that a patient's dentures no longer fit. This can cause a speech problem that is easily cured by a dentist. Sometimes the reduced speech intelligibility is due to something as simple as forgetting to put in dentures. Often speech can be improved by stabilizing dentures with a denture adhesive.

Voice Problems

Following stroke or head trauma, some patients develop weakness or paralysis of the vocal cords. The immediate problem with these patients is to maintain an adequate airway. In severe cases tracheostomy could be required to sustain life.

The voice problems associated with vocal cord weakness or paralysis can vary from a mild breathy "whispering" voice to an inability to produce any sound.

The same suggestions given for communicating with dysarthric patients work well with these patients.

Patients with laryngeal dysfunction should be referred to an otolaryngologist.

Laryngectomy

The patient whose larynx has been removed has lost the ability to produce speech sounds in the normal way. These patients should be given a pad and pencil for transmitting messages. Gestures can also convey information. They should be discouraged from using whispered speech to avoid establishing a habit that will interfere with learning to use esophageal speech.

Aphasia (Input-Output)

This is, perhaps, the most dramatic of the communication impairments encountered by a nurse. Aphasic patients might have nothing wrong with their ears or their speech muscles. They can see and hear and produce sound and still be unable to communicate.

Aphasia is defined as the reduction or loss of the ability to use language symbols as the result of damage to the language centers in the brain. The most familiar language symbol is, of course, the spoken or written word. The patient will have difficulty using words in speaking, listening, reading, and writing. The degree of impairment can range from a mild word-finding problem to loss of ability to communicate in words. In extreme cases the patient will not be able to understand gestures or other symbols.

Damage to the language centers is usually caused by traumatic head injuries or cerebral vascular accidents. The language processes are controlled in almost all cases by the left hemisphere of the brain. Aphasia can occur in the absence of any motor impairment, but it is frequently associated with right-sided motor weakness or paralysis as the left hemisphere controls the right side of the body.

Aphasia usually affects all language modalities—understanding speech, reading, speaking, and writing—although one area can be more severely impaired than the others. Often the ability to understand will be more intact than the ability to speak. However, both are usually affected. This affliction is typically accompanied by a reduction in auditory retention span. For example, a patient may respond to "sit down" but be unable to comprehend "come over here and sit down on this chair." Aphasia is frequently complicated by dysarthria, hemianopsia, reduced attention span, memory impairment, and emotional lability. Fatigue reduces performance.

Communicating with aphasic patients taxes the ingenuity of any nurse. Each patient is different, and even the same patient can vary in his performance from hour to hour or day to day. There are no simple methods that work with all patients, but it is extremely important that you *first determine the patient's level of comprehension and expression.* A patient's smile in response to a communication will often mislead a nurse into thinking that the patient understands. To avoid incorrectly evaluating a patient's communication capability you should ask him to perform a task like, "Touch your nose." Do not gesture! If he does not understand, then use gestures or written words in an attempt to open up avenues of communication. If the patient understands but cannot express himself in other than a "yes" or "no" fashion, you might play twenty questions with him. That is, move from broad to specific questions. With the patient whose primary difficulty is comprehending speech, try reducing speech to short units supplemented with gestures or pantomime. With the patient whose difficulty is expressing his needs, use questions that require a yes or no nodding response. Encourage the patient to point or pantomime, or provide a communication picture book and have him point to the appropriate picture.

Allow plenty of time for a response of any type. Above all, be patient and expect frustration! These patients have a tremendous desire to convey their message and are doing the best they can with the skills available to them at that moment. If all attempts fail, try to reassure the patient that you will try again later.

Basic Techniques

Interference in the communication process can stem from many causes. Confusion and disorientation, hearing loss, visual loss, aphasia, and/or dysarthria following cerebrovascular accident or head injury, loss of voice due to involvement or removal of the larynx, and respiratory insufficiency are among the problems frequently encountered in a hospital. Regardless of etiology, the following techniques should make communication between nurse and patient easier:

1. Speak slowly and distinctly in a normal voice.
2. Use short, simple phrases. A reduced memory span is often a problem in brain-damaged and elderly patients. This does not mean "talking down" to the patient. Treat adult patients as adults.

3. Ask direct questions that can be answered with a simple "yes" or "no." "Does your leg hurt?" rather than "Tell me where it hurts."

4. Give one instruction at a time, and wait for a response before continuing. "Stand up" instead of "Stand up, turn around, and sit on this chair."

5. Repeat questions and instructions, rephrasing to clarify meaning.

6. Supplement speech with gestures and demonstrations if patient appears not to understand.

7. Stand in good light and make sure the patient can see your face. Hard of hearing patients (and many elderly people have a hearing loss) need to supplement auditory input with speech reading.

8. Give instructions to hemiplegic patients from the nonaffected side. These patients sometimes ignore stimuli on the affected side.

9. Use writing and pictures when speech is not effective. Some patients will follow written instructions or understand picture cues.

10. Allow plenty of time for the patient to respond. *This is very important!* Brain-damaged and some elderly patients often need extra time to formulate a response. Conditions of hurry and stress reduce their ability to communicate. Nothing is more frustrating to a person than to try to respond while his questioner is rushing on to a new topic. Encourage the patient to use nonverbal responses such as nodding, pointing, and pantomime if speech and writing abilities are impaired.

Remember! *Communication is a basic human need.* The exchange of ideas and information enables us to relate to other people and to control our environment. Any impairment results in frustration, inadequacy, and a reduced feeling of self-worth. One who shows sympathetic concern and understanding and who exerts the extra effort necessary to improve communication will greatly reduce the fears, depression, and withdrawal behavior of the communication impaired patients.

Posttest for Techniques to Facilitate Communication

Please complete or answer the following statements and questions.

1. *You have just been assigned to work with an aphasic patient. Before you establish a method of communicating with him you should first _____*

2. *If a patient does not understand your spoken words you might try communicating by: ____ _____ or _____*

3. *Your patient has a communication problem. What is wrong with telling him to, "Get up out of the wheelchair, turn toward the window, and sit down on the bed"?_____*

4. *Dysarthria is _____*

5. *With a patient that is hard of hearing you might be able to communicate by using _____ _____ cues.*

6. *Laryngectomy patients should be discouraged from using whispering speech. True or False?*

7. *Your patient has a communication problem resulting from brain damage. He does not respond immediately to your questions. This is because he does not understand you. True or False?*

Answers: Compare your answers with the following:

1. *Determine his level of understanding and communication.*

2. *Writing; pantomime.*

3. *There are probably too many instructions being given at once—these patients usually have a reduced retention span.*

4. *A reduction in speech intelligibility resulting from impairment of the muscle controlling the speech structures.*

5. *Visual.*

6. *True.*

7. *False. He may understand but might require a long time to formulate an answer.*

If you got them all correct, great! If you missed a few, you should review this chapter until you understand the information.

Suggested Readings

American Heart Association. *Aphasia and the Family,* New York, 1969.

Berry, Mildred, and John Eisenson. *Speech Disorders.* New York: Appleton-Century-Crofts, 1956.

Darley, F.L.; Aronson, A.E.; and Brown, J.R. *Motor Speech Disorders.* Philadelphia: W.B. Saunders Co., 1975.

Davis, Hallowell, and Silverman, S. Richard. *Hearing and Deafness.* New York: Holt, Rinehart and Winston, 1960.

National Society for Crippled Children and Adults. *An Open Letter to the Family of an Adult Patient with Aphasia.* Chicago.

Sarno, John E., and Martha T. *Stroke.* New York: McGraw-Hill, 1969.

Schuell, H.; Jenkins, J.; and Jimenez-Pabon, E. *Aphasia in Adults.* New York: Harper and Row, 1969.

Taylor, Martha L. *Understanding Aphasia, A Guide for Family and Friends.* New York: Institute of Rehabilitation Medicine, 1958.

Waldrop, William F. and Gould, Marie. *Your New Voice.* New York: American Cancer Society, 1969.

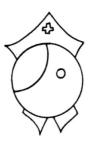

Psycho-Social Aspects of Rehabilitation

JANE JESTER, M.S.W.

4.

Introduction

The basic skills that are used in the rehabilitation of patients cover many aspects. The nurse in the urban and rural areas finds that one has to take on various roles and use a variety of skills. This is true whether one is employed in a hospital or in a nursing home setting.

In the process of rehabilitation, the psycho-social aspects of the patient and his family must be considered. Psycho-social aspects involve the patient's housing, financial, and emotional situations. These aspects can affect the patient's hospitalization, family life, and plans after discharge.

Ordinarily the psycho-social aspects of patient care are the social worker's responsibility. Unfortunately, there is not always a social worker available. In this case the role of social worker must be assumed by someone else. Here we are asking you, the nurse, to perform some of the duties of the social worker. It is not our purpose to make you into social workers. But we do want you to borrow certain skills from this field so you are more effective in total patient care.

In learning how to assess the patient's psycho-social aspects, you will be more effective in dealing with the patient as an individual, not just as a stroke or fractured hip. Through the patient assessment you can be effective in identifying and alleviating psycho-social problems; you might find it easier to offer the patient and his family assistance with discharge plans; and you can become a link between the patient and other staff members (especially, the physician). Although it is important that you share the findings of your assessment with the patient and his family, you must reassure them that this information is kept confidential among the staff. This will help in gaining the trust of the patient and his family.

Objectives

The major goal of this chapter is to enable you to assess effectively the psycho-social aspects of the patient and to utilize the assessment to alleviate problems. Specifically, after working through this chapter you should be able to:

1. utilize the patient assessment to evaluate the patient's personal, financial, and environmental resources;
2. recognize the emotional situations that the patient and his family face during, and following, hospitalization;
3. distribute the information from the patient assessment to other staff members who are involved with the patient; and
4. assist the patient and his family in discharge planning, which would include referring them to appropriate resources.

Objective 1

Utilize the patient assessment to evaluate the patient's personal, financial, and environmental resources. Your first task in looking at the psycho-social aspects is to gather information about three specific areas:

1. personal resources,
2. financial resources,
3. environmental resources.

This information should aid your understanding of the resources available to the patient for meeting his particular needs.

The personal resources of the patient focus on his family. You should be concerned with such matters as:

1. Is there a key person in the family who is closest to the patient?
2. Can you involve them in discharge planning?
3. Do they feel responsible for him?
4. Who comprises the patient's family?
5. Do you detect signs of rejection?
6. Do you detect any family conflict affecting the patient's hospitalization and discharge?

All these questions, when answered, could give you a picture of the family's level of stability.

The area of financial resources can be a delicate matter. In questioning the patient and family about finances, your tone of voice is more important than the wording of the question. The patient and family need to be assured that you are interested in all facets of the patient's life that affect his care, hospitalization, and discharge. Finances can definitely have an effect on these factors. Therefore, you should consider the following questions:

1. Is the hospitalization putting a strain on the family's savings?
2. Could this strain continue after discharge?
3. How is the patient covered financially—does he have Medicare, Medicaid, or private coverage?
4. (If applicable) Will the patient return to his job? Are there other job opportunities?

Now, you may feel that as a nurse you should not be involved with the patient's financial concerns. But, if no social worker or anyone else to handle this problem exists, a small effort on your part can be extremely helpful. Someone needs to be aware of the problem! For example, the physician might decide to transfer the patient to a nursing home. This can cost money. But who pays for the care if funds are nonexistent or low? If you have already made yourself aware of any financial problems, you can offer assistance by informing the physician and/or by seeking an alternate plan. The question of alternate plans will be covered at a later point in the chapter.

Finally, you will be concerned with the environmental resources. When you discuss the patient's environment, you will concentrate on his home. Patients can be discharged to their own home, to a nursing home, or to a relative's home. Therefore, you need to determine what type of home is available to the patient after discharge. Will the patient go to an apartment or a home with a family member? Wherever he goes you need to learn certain things about the home. For instance, when the patient requires assistive devices, you would ask the following questions: Is the home suitable for a wheelchair? How wide are the doors, especially the bathroom door? Is there a tub and/or shower? How many? What size home is it? Could a patient with a walker function easily in the home? Generally, you will find that these questions can apply for many rehabilitation problems that you encounter.

You should now have some idea of the questions you can use in assessing the patient's problems. These questions can assist you in formulating other questions. You should then be able to identify the patient's situation.

Test for Objective 1

Now it is time to check your understanding. Read the example and complete the exercise which follows.

Example: Mary T. is 24 years old and single. She is hospitalized after a car accident which left her a possible paraplegic. The accident occurred while she was on vacation. Her BCBS insurance coverage is through her employer. She is an executive secretary and has worked for two years. Before the accident Ms. T. was earning around $700 monthly. Her mother is deceased, and her father is a farmer living in a small rural town. Ms. T. lives in a large city in an upstairs apartment in a complex near her job. The remainder of her family—two sisters and one brother—is scattered over the state. At the time of her accident, Ms. T. was making plans to be married. Ms. T. has been active in her community serving as a hospital volunteer and attending activities at a Methodist church near her apartment.

Do the exercise below before proceeding.

1. *List the three basic areas of patient assessment. For each area, summarize the appropriate information from the example you just read.*
   a. _____
   b. _____
   c. _____
2. *Again, list the three areas of patient assessment. For each area, list questions which might be used to elicit the information you summarized in No. 1.*
   a. _____
      _____
   b. _____
      _____
   c. _____
      _____

Answers:

1. a. *Personal: father, fiancé, two sisters, one brother, active in community affairs; church work.*
   b. *Financial: employed as executive secretary, salary $700, BCBS insurance through employer.*
   c. *Environmental: from small rural town, lives in large city, lives in upstairs apartment.*
2. a. *Personal: Who comprises patient's family?*
      Who is closest to patient?
   b. *Financial: What insurance is being used? What type of work?*
   b. *Environmental: Where does she live?*
      What type of housing?

If you generally agreed with these answers, move on! If not, think about this a little longer. Sometimes a second try is instructive. You need an understanding of the patient assessment to offer assistance to the patient, family, and staff.

Objective 2

Recognize the emotional situations that the patient and his family face during and following hospitalization. The patient and/or family will find themselves confronted with problems on all sides. We have discussed the personal, financial, and environmental problems that can arise: Now we need to consider the emotional side of illness and disability.

The physical illness suffered by the patient is accompanied by emotional problems. Generally speaking, almost all physical illnesses will have emotional aspects, though they will range from severe to nonsevere. Both the patient and family experience emotional problems, just as they experience the physical illness.

Some of the emotional problems that confront the patient and family include:

1. fear, anxiety, and depression;
2. denial of illness and disability;
3. rejection of the patient by the family, or rejection of the family by the patient.

Now, we will discuss each emotional problem, tell you what it is, and how to handle it.

Fear

In terms of fear, the patient and family might fear what has happened and what could happen. They might be afraid of the future and could be wondering what will happen next. The patient and family can become angry over the illness or disability. They might question: Why has this happened and how? They sometimes look for something or someone on which to place blame.

Anxiety is also experienced by the patient and family. They might worry about legitimate problems or about things with which they should not be concerned. Sometimes they might even create problems. Naturally, when the patient is ill he is not at his best. He lies in bed and has time to think about his situation. If he is a stroke patient, he worries about walking or about speaking. He becomes depressed over his physical situation. Family problems, such as money or marital trouble, might make things worse. It is important, as previously indicated, that you be aware of the patient's total situation. Then, learn to recognize reasons why the patient can become depressed.

A patient who is depressed is usually unmotivated and wishes to be left alone. In a cancer patient, for example, this attitude can be expressed as a wish to be left alone to die. On the other hand, I am sure you have had patients who seemed to complain about everything. If you examined them closely, you would find that the chronic complainer is usually a depressed patient. He is probably unable to express his feelings in any way other than by complaining. The patient is hurting physically and emotionally.

You are probably wondering what you can do to help the depressed patient. We know that recovery from the illness can help to alleviate this condition. But when the patient is still hospitalized, you need to concentrate on understanding both patient and family: Take the time to listen to them. This will make you more aware of the situation. Your patient can be helped by talking things out. This requires having someone with whom he can talk. Patients and families need much assurance about their situation. It is not giving false hope to let them know you feel things might work out and that you are there to help them. It is also important that you control your emotions and keep a positive outlook. Do not become so overly involved in the patient's problems that you cannot help him.

Denial

Denial is the mechanism by which the patient and family avoid reality and cope with a difficult situation. This mechanism becomes unhealthy when it hinders adequate functioning of the patient within his limits and within the future planning of the family.

In working with your patients you will find those who cannot accept their illness or disability. Many times not even the family can accept it. The denial of illness can be very subtle. For instance, the stroke patient could work very hard to walk and be very motivated to get out of bed. When questioned about his motivation, he might comment, "I have to work hard to get my leg well like it was before and get rid of this brace." This patient might always need to wear a brace, yet he cannot accept the reality of the situation. Instead, he seems to be operating with an unrealistic frame of mind. He should concentrate on what life will be like from now on, not as it was in the past.

Family members are also caught in the denial game. A husband may not be able to accept illness in a wife because he would be faced with more responsibility and possible role changes in the family. This would be true especially if the wife were disabled. She might not be able to return home. The family would have to accept and plan for this. When the family continues to deny the disability, this hinders realistic discharge planning.

You should be looking for denial when you have those first contacts with the patient and family. Knowing about denial can give you clues as to how other problems, such as discharge planning, can be handled.

Denial can be a difficult emotional problem to handle. However, there are some helpful techniques which you can use. One technique is to approach the situation as the "reality person" for the patient and family. A "reality person" is one who knows the real situation and acts as a guide for the family and patient.

Other staff members can be involved in handling denial. Sometimes the physician just has to give the family the real aspects of the situation. At other times you can just ignore the patient's denial and continue working with him. Do not let denial hinder your work with the patient. Continue to work within the realm of reality. Sometimes there seems to be nothing you can do. The family could continue to deny that mother needs a nursing home and want to take her back home. In working with this family, you would need much understanding and patience. You have to realize that people function differently and cope with emotional problems differently.

Rejection

Illness and disability can produce feelings of rejection. There can be rejection of the patient by the family, or rejection of the family by the patient.

Many times through lack of understanding of the illness or disability, the family rejects the patient. This rejection does not have to be obvious. For instance, although the patient might not be an invalid, the family treats him as such. This can be a latent form of rejection. The family is sometimes settling for less than what the patient is capable of doing.

There are more apparent ways in which the family might reject the patient. Patients are often placed in nursing homes even when there is no need. Excuses are always given and the truth seldom revealed. Other times, families like the idea of the patient being hospitalized. Grandmother's room at home is transformed into a sewing room. The family acts as if grandmother will be in the hospital eternally.

On the other hand, the patient can reject his family. Because of illness or disability, he develops a low self-image. You begin to see the patient withdraw to his own world. He does not want to participate in family affairs or see anyone. The patient feels bad about himself; therefore, he thinks everyone else feels bad about him.

The patient not only can reject his family, he can also reject himself. He becomes unmotivated, feels worthless, and begins to lose his self-respect. Patients can feel embarrassed about asking for help and being dependent.

Handling rejection calls again for you to act as a "reality person." You must attempt to bring the patient out of his withdrawal. You can engage him in a conversation about a hobby or current events. You can give him emotional support in helping him regain his self-respect. Constant assurance together with encouragement is important. Point out what is good about the patient in terms of his progress. When the patient is able, dressing in street clothes can help him to feel "alive" again. Sitting in the wheelchair and maneuvering around the room can give him a feeling of independence. Try to assure the patient that there is no crime in needing help once in awhile.

The family's rejection of the patient can be handled in much the same way. You can attempt to involve the family in care of the patient. Show them things he can do for himself. Encouragement is important and families need this too. Education of the patient and family about the illness and disability is another way to handle rejection.

The emotional problems we have just considered are interrelated. For example, the patient might deny the disability and, thus, the family would refuse to help him. Or, a patient who is rejected might become depressed.

Remember that you can expect to see all these emotional problems to some degree in your patients. Thus, it is imperative that you be able to recognize and deal with them. The patient's motivation to improve or his will to live are affected by his emotional condition. You have to concentrate on his physical and emotional problems.

Test for Objective 2

Now it's time for another exercise. Read the examples and complete the exercises which follow.

Example No. 1: Ms. T. has been hospitalized for several months. The physician has been working to prepare her for further hospitalization with rehabilitation in mind. The final diagnosis is paraplegia. Ms. T. has been told she will not walk again. The physician is encouraging her to continue therapy to stabilize her function from a wheelchair. Ms. T's thinking has been verbalized as "therapy is important because I have to learn to walk again." But progress is slow. Ms. T. appears less cheerful and optimistic. She has begun to complain about the smallest thing. She seems to have lost interest in her appearance. Also there seems to be lack of desire to think about future therapy. Ms. T. has been acting different toward her father and fiancé each time they visit. The fiancé still has plans for marriage, but Ms. T. has not been willing to discuss this.

Exercise: List three emotional difficulties experienced by Ms. T. For each one list the clues found in the example which provide evidence that an emotional problem exists.

a. _____

b. _____

c. _____

Example No. 2: Ms. T., age 24, is being prepared for discharge to a rehabilitation center for further therapy. But before going to the center there has been some talk about going home for a brief stay. She is undecided about what to do. She has been worried about her financial situation, her job, and apartment. Also, she is still using a catheter. Her marriage plans are indefinite since she has had difficulty in deciding what to do.

Exercise: List the factors that would be important to consider when planning Ms. T's discharge.

_____

_____

_____

_____

Answers: Compare your answers with these:

Exercise No. 1

a. Fear, anxiety, and depression.
b. Denial of illness—disability.
c. Rejection.
Fear, anxiety, and depression—less cheerful and optimistic, complaining, unmotivated.
Denial—learning walking all over again.
Rejection—unmotivated, loss of interest in appearance, changed attitude toward family.

Exercise No. 2

Housing—patient lives in upstairs apartment, which is not too practical.
Apparent emotional problem, involving fiancé, could need counseling. Finances could be a problem if insurance doesn't cover therapy. There is the purchase of equipment.

If you generally agreed with these answers, proceed. If you did not, please review this section before continuing.

Now you should have an idea of what emotional problems the patient and family will have. Your recognition of these problems can help to speed up the patient's recovery and progress.

Now begin reading about how you can involve other staff members with the patient and family.

Objective 3

Distribute the information from the patient assessment to other staff members involved with the patient. For the information you gather in the patient assessment to be effective, it must be utilized. The information should be used to give insight into the patient's total situation. It is important that you have a picture of the whole person including the medical and psycho-social aspects of the situation. Because the patient is in a medical setting, the staff members will already have a medical evaluation. But of equal importance is the psycho-social picture, which you can provide. By disseminating this information to the staff, you are contributing to the patient's rehabilitation. Patients can be difficult, dependent, and unmotivated. Oftentimes, when we have an idea of the patient's family and environmental situation, we have more patience and tolerance toward him. We are more prone to offer emotional support and understanding to the patient.

By being aware of the emotional problems centering around illness, the staff members can better accept the patient's behavior. They become better equipped to handle emotional setbacks. Patients become depressed and apathetic. For the staff to deal with this, they must be aware of and understand these emotional problems.

Information about a patient's emotional problems can be disseminated through personal contact among the doctors and nurses who are directly involved with the patient's care. This information should be recorded in the nurse's notes and on the patient's chart. For example, under Medicare the patient may have a limited time in which he can be hospitalized without undue concern about financial resources. The information you give on the financial resources assists the staff in planning the medical treatment.

By knowing about the problems in the environmental situation, the patient may be taught certain skills that would allow for his return to the home instead of to a nursing home. Long hospitalization can often cause dependency in certain patients. They begin to make their hospital room home. If you are aware of this problem appearing in your patient, you can alert the physician. Thus, this problem can be alleviated before it is allowed to grow.

Test for Objective 3

Now let's see if you understand the above material. Listed below are True-False items. Place T or F beside each statement.

___ 1. *You should tell only the doctor what you learn about the patient.*

___ 2. *Sharing information with others is not really an important way to help your patient.*

___ 3. *If you realize the patient has psycho-social problems, it is important that you should provide a psycho-social picture of him.*

___ 4. *Staff members are better equipped to handle emotional problems when they understand what they are.*

___ 5. *The patient should only be viewed from the medical evaluation.*

___ 6. *The doctor needs to be alerted to financial problems.*

___ 7. *It is hoped that by understanding the patient's psycho-social problems, the staff members will have more patience with him.*

Check your answers:

1. *False.*   5. *False.*
2. *False.*   6. *True.*
3. *True.*   7. *True.*
4. *True.*

We hope you made 100 percent on this exercise. If not, read the information over. Give the questions another go. Then, move ahead to the next section.

Objective 4

Assist the patient and his family in discharge planning and referrals to appropriate sources related to the specific problems.

In this last section, we will give you information that you can use in helping the patient and family with discharge plans. This is another area where you will use the information gained in the patient appraisal. Knowledge of emotional situations will also be helpful here.

Discharge planning should begin as soon as possible after the patient enters the hospital. The family should begin to think about the various choices they may have. These can always change as a patient improves and progresses. The important thing is that the plans must be realistic. You can help here by keeping informed of the patient's medical situation, which could necessitate discussion with the physician about his expectations for the patient. In turn, this can be discussed with the family in terms of how the medical situation affects the discharge plans.

Involvement with the patient should have made you aware of the financial situation. This will help in guiding the family in their plans. Nursing home placement could be a choice for the patient, and it can be expensive. If the patient qualifies he can apply for Medicaid, which would help with the expense.

Then again, the patient might have to go home, although he requires more care than the family feels they can give. Being informed of home health agencies in your area can help here. You might have a city or county health department to which you can refer the family for a visiting nurse. Your community might have a Visiting Nurse Association. In addition, teaching the family a home program regarding the patient's care can be useful.

If the patient goes back to his home, there could be adjustments that need to be made. For example, a ramp might need to be added. If you are aware of the patient's physical environment early enough, you can suggest that such changes be made before discharge.

In the area of discharge planning, it is important that you make yourself aware of what agencies and resources are available to give aid. Knowledge of financial problems can lead to referring the family to the state Department of Public Welfare and the Social Security Office. To understand what benefits exist for patients, you can order handbooks from these offices. For example, some patients might be able to work. You can then refer them to the rehabilitation commission in your area for job counseling and financial assistance. Be aware of city, county, or state services available to your patients. You can write to these various agencies and request the necessary forms required for gaining assistance. For example, most county health departments will require a physician's orders before sending out a nurse. They usually have a form that the physician can complete and mail back to them.

If your town has a Chamber of Commerce, check with them to see about other agencies that could help the patient and family. Your town could have a family service organization to which you could refer the family for help with the emotional problems.

Remember that in discharge planning you are acting as a resource person for the family. You need to be knowledgeable of what your community offers. This is just another way of helping the patient and family.

For your convenience we have listed several referral sources:

1. American Heart Association
2. American Cancer Society—Reach to Recovery
3. Check the yellow pages of your telephone book under "Social Services"
4. Central office of United Fund Division— Community Chest
5. Home health agencies: City Health, County Health, Visiting Nurses Association
6. State Department of Public Welfare
7. Social Security Office
8. Rehabilitation Commission
9. Chamber of Commerce

You become involved in counseling with the family almost daily. Thus, discharge planning is a vital part of the patient's hospitalization. If there is improper planning, the patient can leave the hospital with feelings of uncertainty about which direction to go. Progress he gained in the hospital can be lost if plans were not made and the family was not informed about what is available.

We do not promise that all the problems you encounter will be solved by our suggestions. But, we do feel that the suggestions will apply for some of the problems you handle.

Test for Objective 4

Now complete the following:

1. List two possible sources for home health services:
   a. _____
   b. _____
2. List two possible sources for financial assistance:
   a. _____
   b. _____

3. Answer by circling the appropriate letter(s). Your role centers around the following function(s):
   a. Resource person for the family.
   b. Guiding the family in realistic planning.
   c. Teaching the family.
   d. All of these.
   e. None of these.

Here are the answers—Check yours! (For No. 1 and No. 2 several answers are possible.)

1. a. County Health.
   b. City Health.
2. a. State Department of Public Welfare.
   b. Social Security.
3. d. All of these.

Posttest for Psycho-Social Aspects of Rehabilitation

Answer by placing T (true) or F (false) beside each statement.

_____ 1. The nurse should rarely be concerned with a patient's emotional adjustment to a physical disability.

_____ 2. Information regarding the patient's home environment plays a vital part in determining his plans for discharge.

_____ 3. Families can reject the patient just as patients can reject families.

_____ 4. Long hospitalization does not tend to cause dependency in patients.

_____ 5. Listening to the depressed patient talk out his problems is as important as taking his vital signs.

_____ 6. Information learned regarding the patient's family problems should be shared with the physician and other professional staff.

_____ 7. Due to disability, a patient can develop a low self-image.

Circle the correct answer for the following statements.

8. Psycho-social aspects of the patient's situation would include:
   a. Housing.
   b. Finances.
   c. Emotional problems.
   d. (a) and (c).
   e. All of these.

9. The following are considered emotional problems connected to physical illness:
   a. Fear.
   b. Rejection.
   c. Depression.
   d. Denial of disability.
   e. All the above.

10. The following would be community agencies to which the patient can be referred for assistance:
    a. County Health Department.
    b. Family Service Center.
    c. State Department of Public Welfare.
    d. (a) and (c)
    e. All of these.

Answers: Compare your answers with these:

1. False.
2. True.
3. True.
4. False.
5. True.
6. True.
7. True.
8. e.
9. e.
10. e.

If all your answers are correct, you have a good understanding of the material presented in this chapter. If you missed any, you should review the material until you understand the correct answer.

Suggested Readings

Garrett, Annette. *Interviewing: Its Principles and Methods,* New York: Family Service Association of America, 1942.

"Family-Centered Social Work in Illness and Disability: A Preventive Approach." Monograph VI. New York: National Association of Social Work, 1961.

Pamphlets published by the American Heart Association: "Facts About Strokes." New York: AHA, 1969; "7 Hopeful Facts About Stroke." New York: AHA, 1969; "Aphasia and the Family." New York: AHA, 1969; and "Strokes—A Guide for the Family." New York: AHA, 1969.

Sarno, John E. and Martha Taylor. *Stroke: The Condition and the Patient,* New York: McGraw-Hill Book Company, 1969.

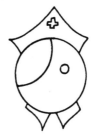

Self-Care Training for Patients with Hemiplegia, Parkinsonism, and Arthritis

RUTH AVIDAN, O.T.R.

5.

Introduction and Objectives

As the patient is engaged in his self-care activities under the supervision and care of the nursing personnel, you will have a direct effect on his attitude and performance. To contribute to the patient's maximal independence, it is of utmost importance that you understand the value of self-care training, have knowledge of the different self-care techniques, and know how to apply them.

Suppose you had a patient who was physically handicapped or mentally confused and couldn't attend to his personal needs:

1. Would you feed, shave, and dress him so he would be comfortable and content? or,
2. Would you evaluate the patient's potential, teach him the proper techniques and encourage him to do as much as he can for himself?

Under the first approach the patient assumes a passive role. He realizes that you, too, have given up hope. Consequently, he will slowly slip into a dependent, depressing, and debilitating existence. Once this existence is established, it becomes very difficult or even impossible to teach the patient self-care activities. The second approach, however, will give the patient a chance to learn to adjust to his disability by spending his energy on things that he can change toward a goal of reaching his own maximal independence. The level of independence attained is limited only by his physical, emotional, and mental deficits.

The self-learning units in this chapter describe eating, personal hygiene, and dressing techniques as they apply to three common diagnoses, namely, hemiplegia, arthritis, and Parkinsonism. Furthermore, this knowledge can be applied to many other disabilities once the principles are understood. The diagnosis, symptoms, and causes are also of vital importance since they provide us with clues concerning:

1. what the patient will be able to do,
2. how he will do it,
3. the problems to be anticipated,
4. the patient's progress,
5. the precautions to be exercised,
6. an outline of the self-care techniques, and
7. the proper way to approach the patient and his family.

The overall objective of this chapter is to familiarize you with self-care training. Since this chapter is designed to furnish fundamental information on self-care, references are provided at the end of each unit which contain detailed information regarding diagnoses, symptoms, causes, treatment, and self-care devices.

Hemiplegia

It is important that the person who takes care of the hemiplegic patient knows how to help him in his self-care activities. Understanding the residual effects of hemiplegia, the proper way to approach the patient, and using the appropriate treatment techniques will promote the patient's physical, mental, and emotional independence. Review of Chapter 1 is important for an intelligent approach to the techniques discussed here.

Hemiplegia is a very broad subject. This chapter, however, contains only the basic and pertinent information regarding self-care training. This learning material is designed to provide a brief introduction to hemiplegia, to discuss the most common problems relevant to this condition, to guide you through the major training procedures, to expose you to a variety of self-help devices, and to present the proper way to approach the patient.

The objective of this unit is to prepare you in the use of basic techniques and procedures for training hemiplegic patients in self-care activities. Specifically, once you complete the instruction in this unit you should be able to:

1. recognize the problems and limitations of hemiplegic patients and identify possible solutions;
2. select appropriate self-help devices and schedules for their use by patients in eating, personal hygiene, dressing, and activities of daily living; and
3. identify procedures to promote patient independence through the use of positive reinforcement and patience.

Activities

The *training of the right hemiplegic* in self-care activities is based upon:

1. Teaching the patient *one-handed techniques,* which require special procedures and, in some cases, special self-help devices.
2. *Training the nondominant hand.* When there is some neurological recovery in the affected arm, the affected arm is used as an assistive hand, mainly to stabilize objects. With additional recovery, the pa-

tient will be able to use the affected hand for performing tasks that require gross dexterity and coordination. The patient or his family might ask about emphasizing the use of the unaffected arm. The reply should be: it is not known how much recovery in the affected upper extremity will take place. Consequently, if we encourage the use of the unaffected arm in self-care and activities for daily living (ADL) early, the patient will have a chance for utilizing his potential toward a realistic goal and reaching his maximum independence. At the same time the affected arm will be exercised in therapy and/or by the patient himself as needed. *A sling* might be used for the affected extremity. Evidence exists to show that a sling does not promote contractures or retard the return of neurological functioning. A sling may be used:
   a. to prevent shoulder subluxation;
   b. to relieve pain in the arm, especially in the shoulder;
   c. to prevent swelling and deformity, especially in the forearm and hand;
   d. for patients who ignore the affected side or have poor sensation on this side, thereby protecting the arm from hot and sharp objects and from getting it caught on doors, wheelchairs, etc; and
   e. to improve sitting and standing balance.
3. *Communicating mostly by demonstration and gestures* due to the language problems.
4. Consideration of *emotional adjustments* the patient must make.

The patient is most likely to succeed if you break the procedures into small steps, follow a sequence from the simplest to the most difficult, allow plenty of time, assist him before he reaches the point of frustration, and praise every effort and success. The latter is the key for motivation and emotional adjustment.

The *training of the left hemiplegic* will be based upon:

1. Teaching the patient *one-handed techniques.* The principles of right hemiplegia apply to left hemiplegia.

2. Considering *slow learning* due to perceptual impairment. Suggestions for training the slow learner are: (a) use *short and clear* verbal instructions; (b) *slow* the patient down to avoid fatigue, frustration, and mistakes; (c) emphasize *position and directions* in space, i.e., right and left, up and down, in and out, behind and in front, instead of using words as "here" and "there", "more" and "less" and so on; (d) emphasize *body parts* and accompany the instructions by *touch*. For example, as you say "shave your right cheek," be sure to touch the patient's right cheek so the patient can see it and, if he has sensation, feel it.
3. Consideration of *emotional adjustments* the patient must make.

Not all hemiplegic patients will gain full independence in self-care and ADL. But remember, even if a patient is partially independent, these can mean a great deal to him. Let the patient do as much as he can for himself, by himself. Also it is important for a patient to be able to feel comfortable about accepting assistance in activities that are beyond his capabilities.

You have just finished an important section. Let's see if you understand and remember the basic facts. Circle the correct answer to the following statements.

1. *You should wait with self-care training and ADL until the affected extremity gains some neurological recovery. True or False*
2. *Instructions to the left hemiplegic patient should be mainly nonverbal. True or False*
3. *With a deficit in visual perception, the patient will have difficulties performing self-care activities. True or False*
4. *A patient with perceptual problems will be a slow learner. True or False*
5. *You can motivate the patient by doing his self-care activities for him. True or False*

Answers:

1. *False.*   4. *True.*
2. *False.*   5. *False.*
3. *True.*

If you missed any of the questions, please review the section again. If you were correct, begin the next section on eating procedures.

Eating: Teaching Swallowing and Self-Help Feeding Devices

Some very sophisticated systems of teaching swallowing have been described.[1] These may be very helpful, especially in patients with cranial nerve damage. For the majority of patients, however, a few simple measures will make the difference. They are as follows:

1. Soft food firm enough to produce a bolus is easier to swallow than fluids. Pureed food or firm gelatin should be tried before water. If aspiration is a problem, gelatin would be preferred.
2. If a nasogastric tube is in place, it might have to be removed before training can begin. Even residual soreness and swelling can inhibit swallowing for several days. There should be no hurry to reinsert the tube; therefore, fluids are IV justified if necessary.
3. In patients with hemiplegia the food should be placed on the "well side."
4. Food is easier to swallow when placed at the back of the mouth.
5. Allow sufficient time for the feeding.

A very important rule in training is that you follow a sequence of procedures starting with tasks that can be mastered easily. In addition, you should use self-help devices whenever necessary. This will avoid frustrating the patient, motivate him to become more independent, and reinforce the learning process.

The sequence of procedures starts with the easy tasks and ends with the more difficult ones. You will find that you do not need them all for each patient. Start from the level at which the patient functions independently. If, for example, the patient has great difficulty in performing at the simplest level, you should talk with the patient, to decide whether to feed him the entire meal, or, support his arm and hand and guide it to his mouth for the first part of the meal, and then feed him the rest of it. This procedure is recommended if the reason for the weakness is low endurance.

Let us examine some of the eating procedures and devices that will be useful to you in rehabilitating the hemiplegic patient.

1. To prevent the plate from moving while the patient is learning to eat, use a wet

washcloth, a suction cup, or suction holder.* Furthermore, a plate guard or a deep dish will help in getting the food on the utensil and prevent it from falling on the table.*

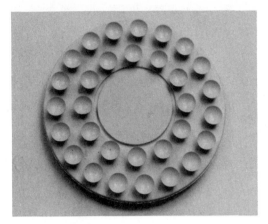

Suction Holder

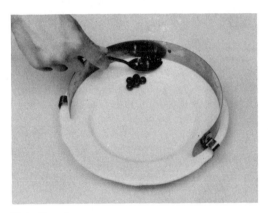

Plate Guard

2. A straw can be helpful if the patient has swallowing problems, poor upper extremity coordination, or weakness. It is good for drinks and clear soup in a cup.
3. It is easier to start with a spoon and solid food such as ice cream, pudding, or applesauce.
4. For a weak grip, a spoon or fork with a built-up handle can be made from a wrapped and taped washcloth around the utensil's handle.*

*These devices can be purchased from Fashion-ABLE and Be OK Self-Help Aids. See sources at the end of the chapter.

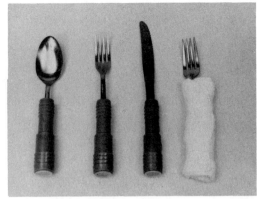

Built-Up Handle Utensils

5. Cutting food with one hand is not easy, but it is possible if you have a sharp knife, tender meat, and the "know-how." To cut the food, hold the knife the way you ordinarily do, placing your index finger on the top part of the blade. Place the tip of the sharp edge on the distant part of the food to be cut, apply pressure on the blade and rock the knife up and down. After each cut, proceed with the tip and repeat the rocking motion until you cut all the way through.

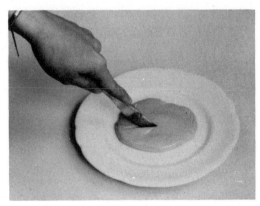

Cutting One-Handed

6. To open jars, stabilize jar by putting it between your knees or place it inside a drawer and lean against it with your hip.
7. To open a carton of milk:
   a. Place the carton so you face the opening side. With your thumb bend each flap all the way back, while your fingers hold the back of the carton.

Self-Care Training for Patients with Hemiplegia, Parkinsonism & Arthritis

b. Then, bend both flaps back at the same time.
c. Push the outer edges of the flap together, thumb against the rest of the fingers, to form a spout.

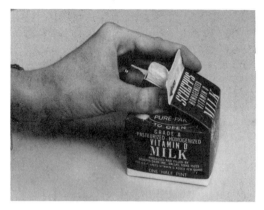

Facing Opening, Thumb on Flap

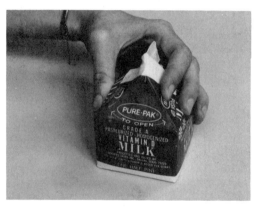

The Two Flaps Pulled Back

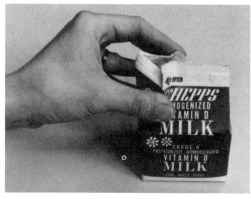

Two Flaps Pushed in to Form a Spout

8. To spread food on bread:
   a. Use soft food from a container.
   b. Grasp handle of the knife with your thumb, the ring, and little finger under (see picture) the handle.
   c. Place index finger on flat side of blade.
   d. Place knife on bread and with middle finger hold bread against the table while spreading the food.

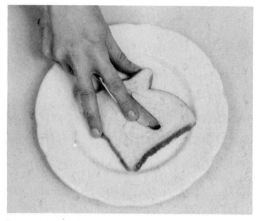

Spreading Food

9. The patient who has hemianopsia might not see the right or left side of the plate. For him to be aware of it, you should tell him that he does not see all the food and show him what he missed. Instruct him to move his head toward the affected side to compensate with the vision that he has. Start by placing the plate on the unaffected side, and gradually with his improved awareness and control over the problem, return the plate to the usual place. Supervision is required.

10. Patients who have severe brain damage are usually mentally confused and might not be able to feed themselves. In addition, even though they may be hungry, they may not be able to relate the food with the necessary action of feeding themselves. To assist the severe brain damaged patient, support the patient's arm under his elbow and around his hand and guide it from his plate to his mouth. With this type of problem, repetition of movements has been found to be effective.

Let's do a quick review of eating procedures and self-help devices by answering the following questions:

1. *After the peas spread all over the table, you realized that you should have used a plate guard. True or False*
2. *The food was too soft and the patient had trouble spreading it on bread. True or False*
3. *To cut food the patient needs an adapted knife. True or False*
4. *For the patient with hemianopsia you should place the food on the affected side and after additional training, place it in front of the patient. True or False*

Answers:

1. *True.*   3. *False.*
2. *False.*   4. *False.*

If any of the answers were incorrect, please review this section again. If your answers were correct, please continue to the next section.

Personal Hygiene Procedures and Self-Help Devices

In completing the section on eating you should have recognized the importance of sequence. Here too, we will start with the tasks that are easy for the patient to perform and learn and finish with the more difficult ones. Remember to instruct or demonstrate each task and then help *only* as much as necessary. The easy tasks will require less help and less practice than the more difficult ones.

1. *Combing hair.* Short hair is easy to handle. Long hair can be kept in place with an elastic band. Patients with hemianopsia and perceptual problems will find it difficult to handle the comb at the back of the head or on the affected side. Since the patient might not know how to use it when you give him the comb, you should instruct him, demonstrate the process, and guide the patient's hand.
2. *Shaving.* The use of an electric razor is preferred for right and left hemiplegia. The electrical outlet should be in easy reach. The patient might neglect to shave the affected side of his face as a result of visual perception problems. Since the patient can have difficulty distinguishing between "right" and "left," "up" and "down," he could be reluctant to shave. In this case, you should let him hold the razor while you guide his hand and give instructions.
3. *Make-up.* Lipstick can be turned out or in by gripping the case between the middle and ring fingers with the base of the lipstick directed upward. Rotate the base using the thumb and index finger. This is not easy and requires practice. There are patients who prefer to put the base of the lipstick between their teeth with the case sticking outside the mouth and then rotate the case with the hand. A powder compact can be glued or attached at the base to a steady surface thus making it easier to open. A woman with perceptual problems or hemianopsia will require supervision and should learn about her deficiencies if she is to reach independence.
4. *Antiperspirant.* With practice a spray can be handled with one hand for both underarms.
5. *Oral Hygiene:*
   a. After meals the patient's mouth should be checked for food accumulated on the affected side, since patients are not aware of that side of their mouth and they might also have severe perceptual problems. Teach the patient to check and clean his mouth after every meal and supervise this activity.
   b. *Use of Toothpaste.* Unscrew toothpaste by holding the tube with three fingers and use the thumb and index

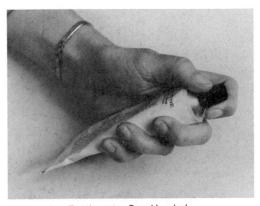

Unscrewing Toothpaste, One-Handed

fingers to screw and unscrew the cap. Some patients may prefer to stabilize the tube gently between their knees and use the free hand to unscrew the cap. Patients with dentures can use an adapted toothbrush with suction cups attached.* Attach the toothbrush to the sink and, grasping the dentures in the hand, brush the teeth. Some patients prefer to rinse their dentures and soak them in denture cleanser.

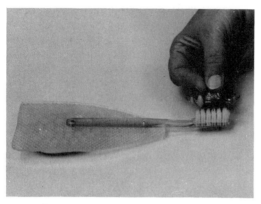

One-Handed Toothbrush for Dentures

6. *Fingernails.* Use a one-handed brush for cleaning nails, and use a file taped onto the table for filing the nails. The affected hand has to be held by the unaffected hand or another file can be used for filing the affected hand on the patient's lap. For toenails use a clipper.

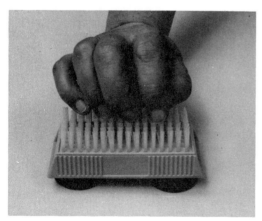

One-Handed Brush for Cleaning Fingernails

7. *Bathing.* The patient should be taught to test warmth of water with the unaffected arm. Always turn on the cold water first and turn off the hot water first. A patient with poor sitting balance will require help when washing lower body parts. Let the patient do as much as he can by himself, but at the same time remember safety. A sponge bath by the sink can be done by the patient with washcloth and long handled sponge and soap on a rope around his neck. The patient should be seated, preferably in a locked wheelchair or an arm chair. In the shower use a steady chair with a back and suction cups attached to its legs. The faucets should be within easy reach. Special equipment for the shower and the tub will contribute to safety. The equipment could include: (a) nonskid tapes on the shower floor, tub bottom, and top edge of the tub; (b) nonslip grab bars attached to the walls at the side of the shower or tub; and (c) a portable shower hose. Do not leave a patient alone when he is bathing unless he is able to function independently.

Now that you have read the above procedures carefully, you should have no trouble answering the following questions:

1. A hemiplegic patient can be trained to become independent in personal hygiene activities. True or False
2. Bathing should be one of the first procedures to be taught. True or False
3. You should praise every effort and every little success. True or False
4. You should encourage the patient to do everything himself, even if it is potentially unsafe. True or False
5. Bathing will require special transfer techniques and special equipment. True or False
6. Inability to recognize the space and part of the body on the affected side because of perceptual problems will affect the learning process and hinder progress. True or False

Answers:

1. *True.*	3. *True.*	5. *True.*
2. *False.*	4. *False.*	6. *True.*

*These devices can be purchased from Fashion-ABLE and Be OK Self-Help Aids. See sources at the end of the chapter.

If you missed any, please review this chapter again. If your answers were correct, proceed now to the next section on dressing procedures.

Dressing Procedures

It is recommended that patients wear street clothing. They should put them on in the morning and wear them for the rest of the day. The patient not only gets the practice dressing this way, but he is also likely to feel less sick, more motivated to learn, and have a more positive attitude toward self-care and getting well. As in personal hygiene, we work on a few dressing procedures simultaneously, still keeping in mind the importance of sequence. We let the patient do more of the easy tasks, and we give additional assistance with the difficult tasks. Eventually, the patient should become independent in the easy tasks and require less help with the more difficult ones. Before we discuss dressing procedures, examine this list of clothing styles that will make dressing easier for the patient:

1. If possible, use clothing that is one size larger than usually worn.
2. Clothes that open completely in the front are preferred.
3. Use dresses, skirts, and pants that slip easily over the hips.
4. Loosely fitting sleeves or armholes as raglan or kimono are preferred.
5. Rayon and nylon jerseys are easier to handle.

All clothing articles including self-help devices should be placed within easy reach of the patient. Now, let's consider the sequence for training the patient to dress himself:

1. *Buttoning and unbuttoning clothes.* On the first day you should explain to the patient that dressing can be done with one hand. Instruct the patient while dressing him so he will become familiar with the procedures. In the early stages let him do the buttoning and unbuttoning, preferably with large buttons. If this presents too many difficulties, let him try a few and you finish. Remember—you do not want to frustrate him.

2. *Putting on a shirt.*
   a. Place shirt on patient's lap with collar toward knees and label showing. Put affected arm across and into the armhole.

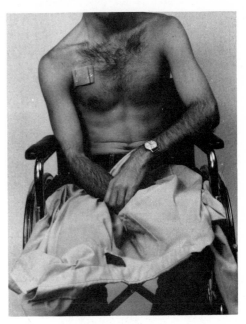

Placing Shirt on Patient's Lap

   b. Pull sleeve up to the elbow and over the affected shoulder. Throw shirt around the back.

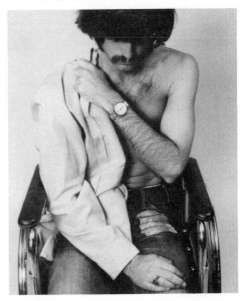

c. Direct the unaffected arm downward and put into the armhole. Button shirt bottom to top. The button of the unaffected hand's cuff should be secured by an elastic thread and kept buttoned at all times. Button cuffs before garment is put on, if the cuffs are wide enough for the hand to get through.

b. Remove sleeve from the unaffected shoulder and work the unaffected arm out of the sleeve.

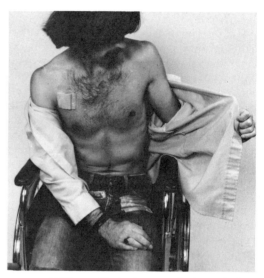

c. With unaffected arm pull sleeve below elbow and then pull off the cuff from the affected arm.

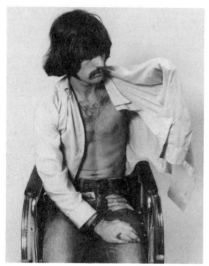

Remember! When you put on a *shirt or a coat,* you put the *affected arm* in first.

3. *Taking shirt off.*
   a. Unbutton sleeve and shirt's front. Push shirt off the affected shoulder using strong hand.

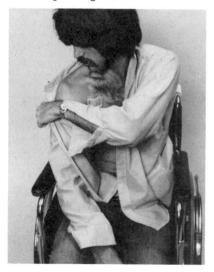

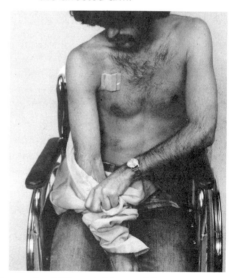

Remember! When *taking a shirt* or coat *off,* the *unaffected* arm comes out first.

4. *Putting on undershirt or slip—Method I.*
   a. Put the affected arm through strap or sleeve by placing the affected arm on

your knee and pulling the strap or sleeve over the hand and up to the elbow.

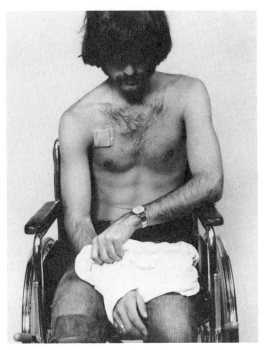

b. Put unaffected arm through strap or sleeve.

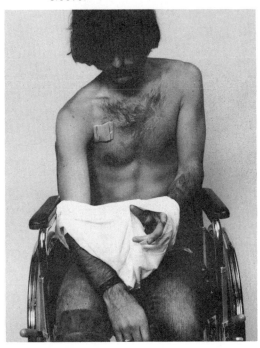

c. The unaffected arm should hold the garment at head opening and slip it over the head and adjust.

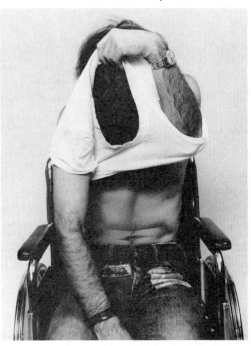

5. *Putting on undershirt or slip—Method II.*
   a. Gather clothing in unaffected arm, and slip over affected arm. Slip over head.

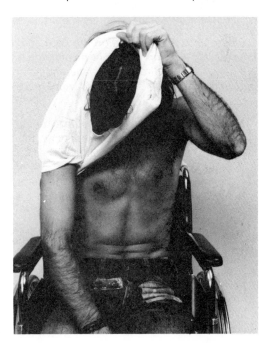

b. Put unaffected arm through strap or sleeve and adjust.

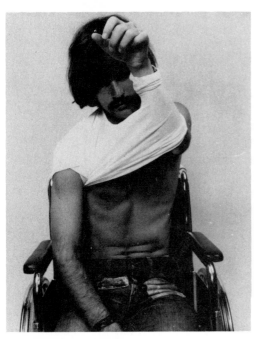

6. *Taking off undershirt or slip.*
   a. With unaffected hand grasping the shirt from the back, pull forward and over the head.
   b. Remove unaffected arm from shirt.
   c. Remove affected arm from shirt.

Please answer this question: You are about to teach Mr. K., who is a right hemiplegic, to put on his undershirt. Which hand should be put in first? If you said right hand, you are correct.

7. *Putting on and taking off shorts, underpants, and slacks.* If the patient has good sitting and standing balance, he can dress while sitting on a regular chair or on the side of a steady low bed. If the patient has poor sitting and standing balance, he should dress while sitting in a locked wheelchair. If the patient is too heavy or too weak, it is easier to dress the lower extremities in bed.

8. *Putting on shorts or pants.*
   a. Sitting down, the patient picks up his affected leg with his unaffected hand and places it over his unaffected leg.

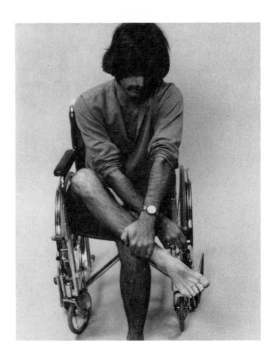

b. Patient holds pants, bends down, and puts the pants on the affected leg.

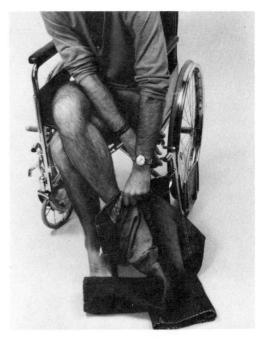

c. Patient uncrosses legs, puts unaffected leg into pants.
d. Patient pulls slacks up to his knees, stands up (with unaffected leg placed

in the midline of the body), and pulls them up by raising the hips, using unaffected leg.

9. *Taking off shorts or pants.* This is done in the reverse procedure, undressing the unaffected leg first.

10. *Putting on bra.*
   a. Panties should be put on first.
   b. Use patient's regular back-fastening bra.
   c. A regular clothespin will be required.
   d. If the patient's right side is affected, place the eyes in front. Use the unaffected arm to fasten bra to panties with clothespin.

e. Pull the other end around your waist with the unaffected hand, making sure that the right side of the bra is out. Hook bra with unaffected hand.

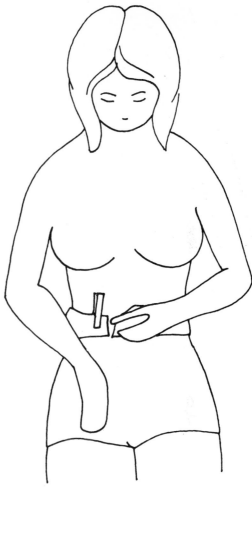

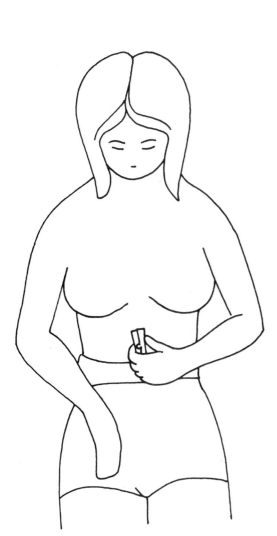

f. Take clothespin off, turn bra around into proper position.
g. With unaffected hand put affected arm through strap and pull up over shoulder.

h. Put unaffected arm through strap and pull strap up.

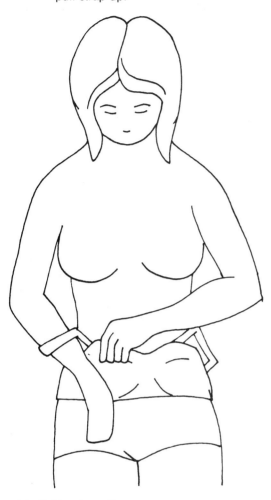

11. *Taking bra off.*
    a. Pull strap off affected shoulder down to the elbow, repeat procedure with unaffected shoulder, and get arm out.
    b. Use unaffected arm to pull affected arm out.
    c. Turn bra around waist so that the hooks are in the front.
    d. Unhook by holding thumb against rest of fingers.

Remember! Have a patient with poor balance sit in a steady armchair or locked wheelchair.

12. *Putting on socks.* (For the hemiplegic it is easier to put on socks than to put on hosiery. A footstool could be helpful.)
    a. Have the patient sit in an armchair or a locked wheelchair. Using his strong

hand, he places the affected leg over the unaffected leg, or places it on a stool.
    b. The top of the sock is opened by placing the hand in the cuff and spreading the thumb away from the rest of the fingers.

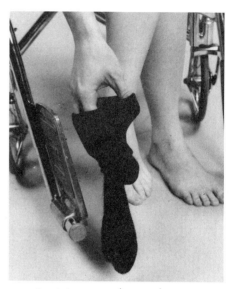

    c. Sock is placed over toes and pulled over foot.
    d. Repeat procedure with unaffected leg. Make sure that there are no wrinkles.

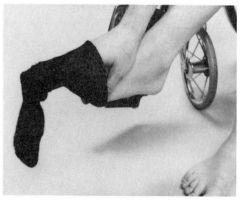

13. *Alternate method for putting on socks.* Again, begin by crossing the legs. Turn the socks inside out, and push the toe part in. Place the toe part over the toes, and pull the sock over the heel and up the ankle.

14. *Putting on and taking off braces.*
    a. Shoes with buckles are easier to handle than those with shoe laces.
    b. Elastic shoe laces are not recommended for spastic feet.
    c. Velcro on the brace's closure is easier to handle than a buckle.
    d. "Insert-A-Foot Shoe Aid"* can be handled easier with one hand than a long shoehorn. This device is slipped over the shoe heel before putting the shoe on. The foot slips into the shoe without effort. When the foot is in the shoe, the device is slipped out.

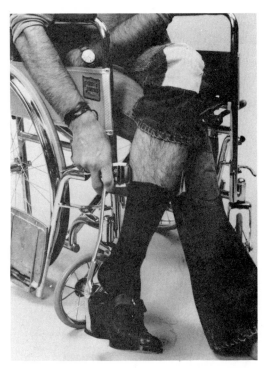

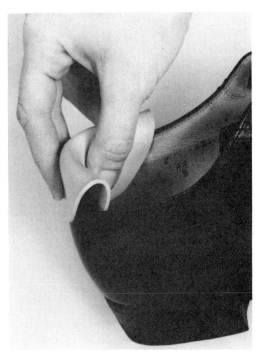

d. With the strong hand put the foot down on the floor and push down on the knee until the heel gets into the shoe.

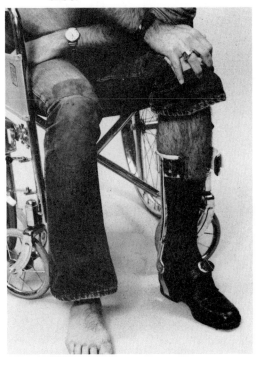

15. *Putting shoes on.*
    a. Sitting down, place the shoe aid over the shoe heel.
    b. With the strong hand pick up the affected leg and place it over the unaffected leg. Hold the shoe and brace by the top of brace. If no brace is involved, hold the shoe tongue.
    c. Place the shoe in front of the leg and slip the foot into the shoe as far as possible.

*Available at Be OK Self-Help Aids or can be made in an occupational therapy department.

e. Pull out the shoe aid and buckle the shoe and brace.

f. Place the shoe aid in the second shoe. Put the shoe on the floor or a stool.

g. Slip the foot in, pull the device out, and buckle the shoe.

16. *Fastening shoe.*

a. *One-handed tying.* This method requires good carryover and good hip flexion to reach the shoe.

One-Hand Bow

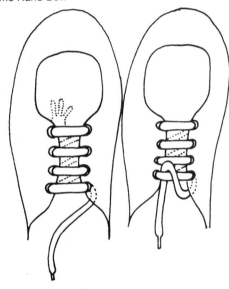

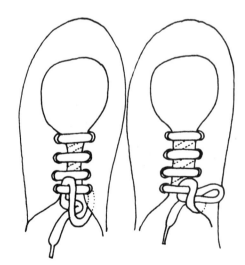

One-Hand Bow

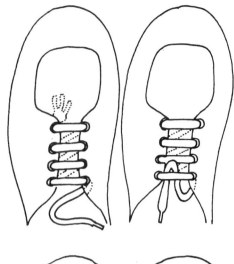

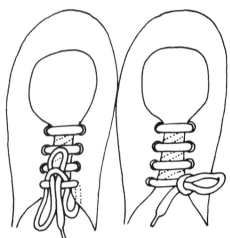

b. Velcro Closures. These are easily made by sewing a 2-inch piece of Velcro loop and a 3-inch piece of Velcro pile together. Then secure it to the shoe by sewing through the eyelets and at the bottom near the

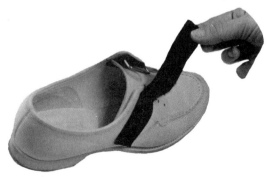

sole. Secure a metal or plastic "D" ring or rectangle to the opposite side with a piece of Velcro sewn through the eyelets.

c. Elastic shoe laces are also available but are not recommended for patients with spasticity.

Let's review dressing procedures by answering the following questions:

1. *A right hemiplegic should put the left hand in first when putting on a shirt. True or False*
2. *Putting on socks is one of the easier tasks. True or False*
3. *When a left hemiplegic takes his pants off, he takes them off his right leg first. True or False*
4. *When Mr. J., a right hemiplegic, took off his coat, he should have taken his left arm out first. True or False*
5. *Mrs. B. has left hemiplegia with poor sitting balance. She should dress mainly from a locked wheelchair. True or False*
6. *Putting on a bra requires a clothespin and a special procedure. True or False*
7. *To put on the brace and shoe, you should cross affected leg over the unaffected leg and place shoe in front of leg. True or False*
8. *Hemiplegics should use a long shoehorn for putting on their shoes. True or False*

Answers:

1. False.	4. True.	7. True.
2. False.	5. True.	8. False.
3. True.	6. True.	

If you missed any of these questions, please review the appropriate material before you proceed. When you are confident that you understand these procedures, continue to the next section.

Activities of Daily Living

In this section, we will discuss briefly some activities that are important for keeping with the patient's interests and for keeping him happy. Activities of daily living include any activity that will promote maximum psychological, physical, social, and vocational independence of the physically disabled individual. The meaning of this term is broad and varied

due to the individual differences of the patients. The ADL are a challenge to your creative efforts to bring about happiness. Furthermore, your knowledge of the basic procedures assures carry-over from the training in the different therapy departments onto the ward.

If, however, you encounter a problem that you cannot solve in this area, refer to the references provided at the end of this chapter or, preferably, contact an occupational therapist.

Reading—A one-handed patient can use a book holder (available at Fashion-ABLE and Be OK Self-Help Aids) or a "book butler" when flat on his back (also available at above).

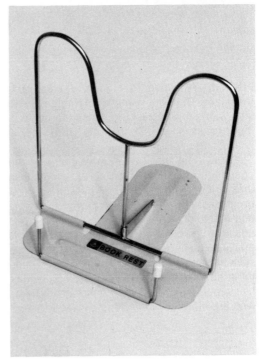

A Book Holder

Following a stroke many patients find it difficult both to handle and read a newspaper. Placing the newspaper on a table might help. Reading titles or small paragraphs would be a good start. There are patients who complain that when they start reading again, after the stroke, the words and lines get mixed up. They get discouraged and give up reading. A piece of white cardboard with a cut-out window can be very helpful. The window exposes one line at a time, and the cardboard is big enough to cover a large portion of the written or printed matter, which eliminates distractions.

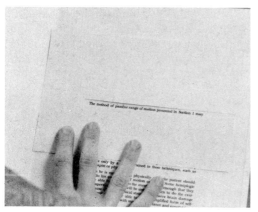

Cut-Out Window

Writing—A clipboard is good for stabilizing the paper. The right hemiplegic might have to start with a felt-tip pen and with some prewriting exercises, e.g., horizontal and vertical lines along the paper, circles, half circles, etc. The prewriting activities improve dexterity and coordination and are easier to accomplish than writing with the left hand. As the patient progresses, he will be able to print his name and eventually write it. After he has developed this skill, you can have him write simple words that are meaningful to him and are in daily use, such as spoon, fork, table, chair, etc. You can tell if he understands those words by asking him to point to objects or to a picture. Patients who are more severely affected need to start

by tracing your prewriting with their finger, then tracing it with a pen. The next stage would be to have them copy your prewriting and, later on, their name. Finally, if the patient's job requires a lot of writing, you should consider training both hands. The patient might develop better endurance and flow of writing in his left hand.

Telephone—A phone amplifier is similar to a two-way loudspeaker, leaving both hands free. It does not require installation or wires. (Available at Fashion-ABLE.)

If the patient has trouble dialing the telephone due to hemianopsia, perceptual problems or language problems, you can help him practice with the receiver down.

Card Playing—A card holder and automatic card shuffler for the one-handed person are available from Be OK Self-Help Aids and Fashion-ABLE.

Sewing—One-handed women should not stop their hobby of embroidery or the tasks of sewing buttons and repairing clothes. Use a simple frame made out of plywood with padded cushions on both ends (stuffed with an old stocking or any other soft material). The horizontal piece should be clamped to a table with a "C" clamp, and the material to be worked on stretched and pinned to the cushions. Sewing is done by working the needle up and down. To thread the needle, stick it in the cushion with the eye up.

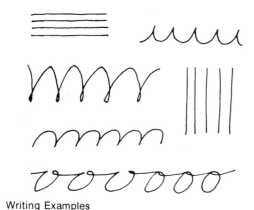

Writing Examples

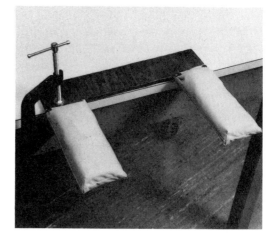

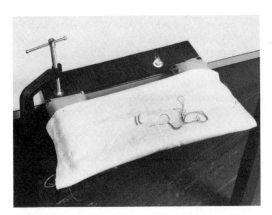

Embroidery Frame

Homemaking and Work Simplifications—
Homemaking and work simplification are very important for disabled women and men, especially for those who have to be at home by themselves and must manage as much housework as possible. There are many techniques, procedures, and pieces of special equipment that the one-handed person can learn to use. Listed below are two excellent references which should be helpful to you.

1. *Mealtime Manual for the Aged and Handicapped*, prepared by the Institute of Rehabilitation Medicine, New York University Medical Center, Essandess Special Editions, a Division of Simon and Schuster, Inc., 630 Fifth Avenue, New York, New York 10020. Available on order or from bookstores. Spiral bound $2.38; paper-on-board $6.49.
2. Your local American Heart Association.

Please answer the following questions for this section:

1. A patient who eats, dresses, and attends to personal hygiene independently will have a better self-image. True or False
2. The self-help device for sewing is expensive. True or False
3. When the patient complains that words and lines get mixed up when he is reading, you should suggest changing his glasses. True or False
4. It does not make sense to train a patient to use both hands in writing if the affected hand is not gaining enough recovery for holding a pen. True or False

Answers:
1. *True.*   3. *False.*
2. *False.*   4. *False.*

Posttest for Hemiplegia

Please circle the correct answer or answers for each item.

1. Hemianopsia can be corrected with prescription glasses. True or False
2. Which of the following are problems associated with right hemiplegia?
   a. Speech disorders.
   b. Paralysis on left side.
   c. Paralysis on right side.
   d. Perceptual problems.
   e. Tremor.
3. The proper sequence in self-care training is important because:
   (choose the correct reasons)
   a. It encourages the patient to become independent.
   b. It reinforces the learning process.
   c. It reduces patient frustration.
   d. It ignores the necessity for teaching simple tasks.
4. Which of the following self-help devices would you select for eating procedures for the left hemiplegic patient?
   a. Fork.
   b. Plate guard.
   c. Built-up spoon.
   d. Suction cup.
5. Which of the following problems might prevent the patient with left hemiplegia from combing the hair on the back of his head?
   a. Limited range of motion.
   b. Perceptual problems.
   c. Poor demonstration.
   d. Patient's confusion.
6. Mrs. K. is a right hemiplegic with severe speech impairment. You are planning to teach her dressing techniques. Which of the following techniques would you use first?
   a. Give her verbal instructions for dressing procedures.
   b. Explain the difficulties in putting on a shirt.
   c. Demonstrate the proper procedures to put on a shirt.
   d. Ask her to put on the shirt.

7. In putting a coat on a right hemiplegic, which extremity would you put in first?
   a. Right.
   b. Left.

8. A left hemiplegic with complete paralysis, hemianopsia, perceptual problems, and unawareness of the body and space on the left will have difficulties with:
   a. Eating.
   b. Speech.
   c. Shaving.
   d. Dressing.

9. Mr. A. will shave today for the first time after his stroke. What would you do?
   a. Ask the orderly to do it.
   b. Give him the electric razor and tell him that you will be right back.
   c. Shave him yourself.
   d. Observe him when he shaves, and help when necessary.

10. A hemiplegic woman will not require help to put on her make-up since she is used to doing it. True or False

11. A right hemiplegic begins to practice writing by writing his name. True or False

12. You notice that the hemiplegic arm is bruised over and over again, and that the hand gets caught in the wheelchair spokes. What would you do about it?
    a. Suggest an arm sling.
    b. Tell the patient to watch for his hand.
    c. Explain to him that he should watch where he is going.
    d. Attach a protective shield to the spokes.

13. Training the patient in self-care takes more time at the beginning of the program and less time after he has had the benefit of some practice and repetitions. True or False

14. Mrs. M. is very particular about her appearance. After assisting her in dressing herself, she asks you to comb her hair and put her make-up on. Would you:
    a. Let her do her best and assure her that you will finish so that it looks right.
    b. Hand her the comb and assure her that she can do a good job of combing her own hair.
    c. Fix her hair and make-up for her but tell her she will have to try to do it next time.
    d. Tell her not to worry about how she

looks. She will eventually be able to do a good job herself.

15. A left hemiplegic is trying to feed himself for the first time. Which of these procedures would you follow?
    a. Give him a plate guard.
    b. Show him how to cut his own meat with a rocker knife.
    c. Prepare his food for him and hand him the fork.
    d. Give him a fork with a built-up handle.

16. Which are the most commonly used devices for dressing:
    a. Clothespins.
    b. Shoe aids.
    c. Elastic shoe laces.
    d. Button hooks.
    e. Stocking cones.

17. Mrs. A. has had a light stroke affecting her right side. She is not aphasic. It is her second day in learning to dress herself. She feels she can not do anything for herself and often refuses to try. How can you best help her?
    a. By refusing to help her with steps you know she can do.
    b. By pointing out what she did the day before and giving her an easily attainable goal for the day.
    c. By dressing her and telling her she will have to try it by herself tomorrow.
    d. By leaving her with her clothes and telling her you will help when she is ready to learn to help herself.

Answers:

1. False.	7. a	13. True.
2. a, c	8. a, c, d	14. a
3. a, b, c	9. d	15. c
4. b, d	10. False.	16. a, b
5. a, b, d	11. False.	17. b
6. c	12. a, d	

If you missed any of the answers, review those sections which were difficult to you. If there are still some confusing facts that have not been explained by this unit, make notes and ask for further explanation during the clinical experience. If, however, you answered all the questions correctly you have accomplished the objectives of this unit.

Arthritis and Parkinsonism

The knowledge that you acquired from the unit on hemiplegia will be useful in teaching self-care to patients with other disabilities since you can apply many of the same dressing, eating, and hygienic procedures and self-help devices. The following unit contains a discussion ot the unique aspects of self-care training of two common chronic disorders, arthritis and Parkinsonism. The additional concepts and technical knowledge learned here are applicable to arthritis, Parkinsonism, and similar disabilities. Specifically, once you complete the instruction in this unit you should be able to:

1. Identify the major disabilities and problems faced by arthritic and Parkinson's patients.
2. Select appropriate self-help devices and schedules for their use by patients in eating, personal hygiene, and dressing.
3. Identify and defend appropriate sequences and procedures for training patients in self-care.
4. Identify procedures to promote patient independence through the use of positive reinforcement and patience.

Arthritis

The word "arthritis" means *inflammation of a joint*. The term "arthritis" is used for many different conditions that cause pain in the joints and connective tissues throughout the body. However, not all of these conditions involve inflammation.

The two most common forms of arthritis are *osteoarthritis* and *rheumatoid arthritis*. We will review both of these very briefly. Then we will discuss the self-care for rheumatoid arthritis since it presents more clinical problems and the self-care techniques can easily be applied to other disabilities such as osteoarthritis, fractured hip, hip contractures, senility, different types of cancer, and general weakness.

Osteoarthritis

Osteoarthritis is a noninflammatory, non-systemic disease. It most often affects the weight bearing joints such as the knees, hips, and spine, but often involves the fingers as well. It is a "degenerative" process that begins in the cartilage. It can deform the joint but seldom is disabling except when far advanced in the hips.

Rheumatoid Arthritis

Rheumatoid arthritis is an inflammatory, systemic, and chronic disease that occurs in three stages: acute, subacute, and chronic. It primarily affects the joints, but can affect the eyes, heart, lungs, spleen, liver, blood vessels, kidneys, and digestive system.

The acute stage of the inflammation of the joints is characterized by the typical symptoms of pain, local swelling, redness, restricted range of motion and, possibly, fluid in the joints. In the acute stage, complete rest is indicated. While in the subacute stage the symptoms begin to subside, and the patient is permitted to function with the upper extremities within the limits of his pain.

In the chronic stages, there are no signs of acute inflammation, but three major disabling factors interfere with functioning:

1. *Pain.* Pain is caused by the inflammation and instability of the joint. The pain can be local or general. The severity of the pain can vary throughout the day and from day-to-day. The pain can exist throughout the three stages and can hinder the patient from functioning. You might find that the patient hesitates to function from fear of pain. Also aching and stiffness result from periods of inactivity.
2. *Joint disorders.* After the acute stage is over, the limited range of motion (ROM) leads to contractures due to adhesions (scarring), and the process can end with complete loss of movement within the joint—ankylosis. Limitation in ROM will result from the ankylosis, subluxation, or dislocation. There is likely to be joint instability, too.
3. *Muscle weakness.* The result of disuse that is caused by the pain and limited ROM.

Review: For a short review, answer these questions:

1. Which of the following are anticipated symptoms in arthritis?

a. Pain.
b. Sensory loss.
c. Paralysis.
d. Muscle weakness.
e. Joint disorders.
2. Rheumatoid arthritis affects primarily the joints. *True or False*
3. Rheumatoid arthritis is a degenerative disease. *True or False*
4. You would encourage independence in the acute stage to ensure a good start. *True or False*
5. A fused joint is the result of inactivity. *True or False*

Answers:

1. a, d, e.
2. True.
3. False.
4. False.
5. False.

If you missed any questions review this section again. If you answered all questions correctly you are ready to proceed to the next section.

Self-Care Training

In self-care training the stage of the disease determines how much the patient should be encouraged to do for himself. The desirable amount of effort to be spent by the patient depends on the joint's condition and his general endurance for pain.

Depending on the functional deficit, many of the procedures and self-help devices that you used for the hemiplegic can be applied to self-care training of the arthritic patient. In addition, there are some supplemental self-care techniques with which you should become familiar. They are:

1. To avoid deformity, emphasize the correct positioning of the body at all times.
2. Emphasize the sequence of self-care procedures. The same concept and procedures you used with hemiplegia apply here with slight changes. These changes will be discussed throughout the remainder of the chapter.
3. Although self-help devices play the most important role in rehabilitating the arthritic patients in self-care and ADL, the devices should be used *only if necessary*

and should be kept to a minimum. The devices are used:
a. to contribute to patient independence in self-care when his ROM is restricted and hinders him from performing the desired activities,
b. to conserve energy, and
c. to avoid stress on involved joints.
4. Stress the use of the proper body mechanics and the simplification of the procedures in the activities of daily living. This will help the patient conserve valuable energy and prevent further damage to the joint.
5. The arthritic patient requires a lot of empathy. You must realize that he faces constant pain, disability, and depression. Encouragement and prodding are necessary to help him become independent. You must learn to determine when to prod and when to comfort the patient since this is the key to maximizing his self-care capabilities and making him happy.

Self-Help Devices for Eating

Since the basic eating procedures are similar to those of the hemiplegic patient, variations in terms of self-help devices and procedures unique to rehabilitating the arthritic patient will be presented in this section. If you would like to refresh your knowledge of basic eating procedures, refer to Self-Care Training for the Patient with Hemiplegia.

1. In limited ROM of the shoulder and elbow, use long-handled, lightweight utensils that can be positioned at any desired angle.*

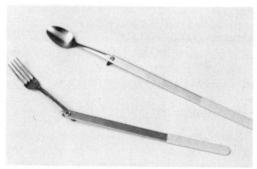

*Available at Be OK Self-Help Aids.

2. In limited ROM of the forearm, use swivel spoon.*

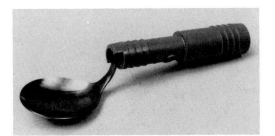

3. If the wrist is painful and unstable, consult with the physician about a wristlet or a wrist splint to reduce pain and stabilize the wrist.
4. In limited ROM or weakness of hand, you may use a:
   a. Universal cuff or utensil holder.*
   b. Built-up handle (see hemiplegic unit).
   c. Interlace utensil holder.*

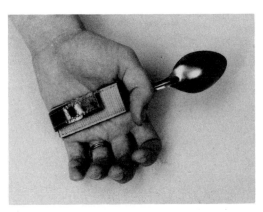

5. For drinking, the patient can use two hands around the cup or a "No Tip Glass Keeper" with a straw holder.* The straw can be stabilized by a pencil clip fastened to a cup.

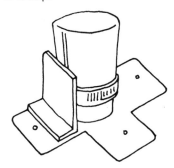

Glass Holder

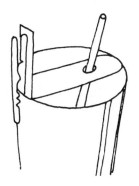

Straw Holder

The patient may refuse to eat in the presence of other people but should be encouraged to do so. If possible sit him with other physically disabled patients who have a positive outlook and attitude. It might help the patient accept the things he cannot change and direct his energy toward more realistic goals.

Self-Help Devices for Personal Hygiene

As you will notice, there is a slight difference in the sequence here, due to the fact that in arthritis, the major problems are limited to ROM and weakness, whereas in hemiplegia, the major physical problem in self-care is the one-handedness. Long-handled devices and special holders are used to overcome the limitation in ROM, to conserve energy, and to avoid stress on the joints.

Temporary extensions can be made by taping a tongue depressor to an object and wrapping with a washcloth. If necessary, this extension can be attached at an angle.

1. *Shaving.*
   a. An electric shaver is preferable. If necessary, it can be provided with a holder for use by a patient with a weak grip.**
   b. A manual razor can be extended with a hollow metal or wooden attachment.
2. *Make-up.*
   a. If the patient has trouble reaching her mouth, the lipstick can be mounted on aluminum tubing.
   b. Use a mirror that can be hung around

*Available at Be OK Self-Help Aids and Fashion-ABLE.
**Available at Be OK Self-Help Aids.

the neck by a plastic loop. These are available at most drug stores.

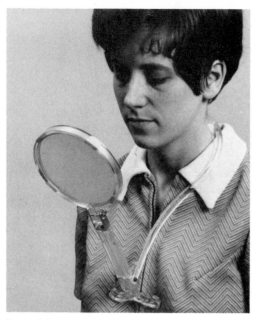
Around the Neck Mirror

3. *Oral Hygiene.*
   a. Use a toothbrush with a long or built-up handle when the patient cannot reach his mouth easily. A regular toothbrush can be modified with an extension.
   b. The toothpaste is not a problem unless the cap is screwed on too tightly.
4. *Combing Hair.*
   a. A long-handled brush and comb can be useful.* These can be purchased or made by adding a wooden attachment.
   b. Short hair is easier to handle.

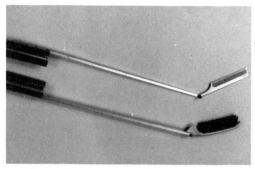
Long-handled Comb and Brush

5. *Fingernails.*
   a. Can be cleaned with a brush which fits over the palmar part of the hand (available at most stores), or a brush that attaches to the sink with suction cups (see Hemiplegic unit).
   b. Fingernails can be filed by using a nail file with a built-up handle made out of cork or a tongue depressor with a washcloth taped around it.
   c. For toenails the patient might require help.
6. *Bathing.* Bathing is among the most difficult tasks in self-care. You should be familiar with transfer techniques and be able to coordinate the patient potential with the proper techniques. (See Chapter 1.) The assistive equipment and devices play an important role for energy conservation and safety. These include:
   a. *Stable chairs* with backs and suction cups attached to the bottom of the legs. One chair beside the tub, another one with shorter legs in the tub. The seats should be even with the edge of the tub. For stronger, lower extremities, a bathtub seat that is adjustable in height would be adequate.
   b. *Nonskid tape* with a rubber surface should be used for the bottom and edge of the tub.
   c. *Grab bars* attached to the walls at the side and head of the tub to hold and push on.
   d. A *portable shower hose.*
   e. A *bathtub safety rail* to assist in getting in and out of the tub.
   f. A *long-handled sponge and brush.***
   g. A *bath mitten* with a pocket for the soap.

A sponge bath by the sink will be the easiest for the patient to handle. The shower is less difficult and is safer to use than the tub.

Review: Answer the following questions:

1. *It's most likely that an arthritic patient will require all the self-help devices mentioned above. True or False*
2. *Generally, the same self-help devices are used for the hemiplegic patients and for the arthritic patients. True or False*

*Available at Be OK Self-Help Aids.
**Fashion-ABLE

3. For limited ROM of the forearm the patient requires a swivel spoon. *True or False*
4. Conserving energy is an important consideration in the arthritis patient's life. *True or False*
5. The arthritic patient will require the long-handled hair brush more often than the long-handled toothbrush. *True or False*

Answers:

1. False.   4. True.
2. False.   5. True.
3. True.

If your answers were correct, you should proceed to the next section on dressing.

Dressing Procedures

1. While dressing, the patient should be seated on a chair with his clothes in easy reach.
2. A stool will help when dressing the lower extremities by making it easier to reach the feet. This saves stress on the spine.
3. If one extremity is not very functional, the hemiplegic techniques should be applied for dressing the upper extremities. To avoid stress on the finger joints, do not use a clothespin when putting on a bra unless it is necessary.

Self-Help Devices for Dressing

1. The same styles of clothing suggested for the hemiplegic patient are suitable for the arthritic patient. The patient's needs will dictate the type of clothing he should wear, whether it be regular clothing, regular clothing with adaptations, or specially designed clothing.
   a. Regular or ready made clothing includes a wide variety of styles, fabrics, sizes, closures, etc. If carefully selected it can save having to make adaptations or buying specially designed clothes.
   b. Adaptation can be done on the patient's own clothes by converting buttons to Velcro or zippers, using elasticized bands for skirts, having dresses open all the way in the front, and by changing zippers in pants to Velcro.
   c. Specially designed clothes with the easy-on and easy-off feature are available commercially at Fashion-ABLE and Vocational Guidance and Rehabilitation Services (see sources at the end of this chapter).
2. Button hooks make buttoning easier and are available in various shapes. To use one, grip the handle, push the wire loop through the buttonhole, catch the button by the wire loop and pull it through the buttonhole. Release the button hook.

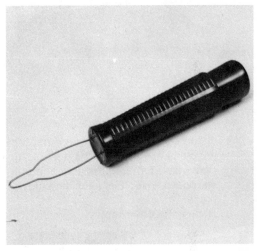

Button Hook

3. A stick with a clothespin taped to the end can be useful when putting on shorts. (Clothespin can be used only when hands are not affected; use hook on stick when hands are affected.) After hooking the clothespin to the shorts, the patient holds onto the other end of the stick while stepping into the shorts. He then pulls them up by means of the stick and unhooks the clothespin.
4. A device is available to aid in putting on stockings or socks. Below are step-by-step instructions on how to use this device:
   a. Sitting in a locked wheelchair or a stable armchair, extend the leg forward or place the leg on a stool.

b. Insert cone up to the toe of the sock.

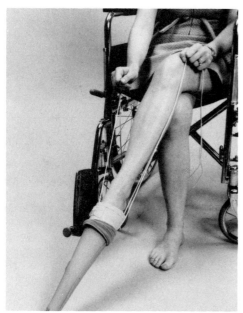

Device to Put on Stockings

c. Guide cone over the toes so that the middle is aligned with the heel of the foot. Insert foot into opening and pull straps up, over the heel, and up in place.

d. Repeat the other foot.

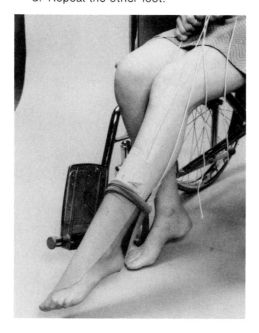

5. To take stockings off:
   Use a long shoe horn to push the stocking or sock off the heel and off the foot. Repeat with other foot.
6. To put on shoes use a long shoe horn as described below:
   a. With the shoe on the floor or on a stool, place the long shoe horn in front of the shoe tongue; put toes in.

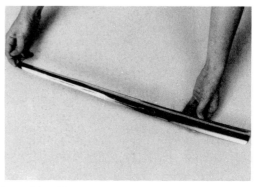

Long Shoe Horn

   b. Now place the shoe horn at the back of the shoe and press down on the knee.
   c. Fasten shoe.
   d. Repeat with other foot.

These procedures are designed to eliminate stress on the back, hips, and knees. The first attempts will be difficult for the patient so be sure to encourage him, and assist him if necessary.

Energy Conservation and Work Simplification

Most energy conservation and work simplification techniques apply to the patient in the home situation and are not among our objectives. Therefore, only a few useful suggestions will be made. The patient in need should be referred to an occupational therapy department.

1. In conversing with the patient you will find that some of his routine activities can be simplified or eliminated. He should *avoid overfatigue* and have frequent, short rest periods during the day.
2. The patient should be instructed in the use of proper body mechanics when sit-

ting, standing, walking, climbing stairs, pulling, lifting, or pushing weight (see Chapter 2).

3. Whenever possible, the patient should avoid lifting, pulling, or carrying heavy objects. A cart, a small table on casters, or any other device with wheels or rollers should be used. These aids should be used for food, dishes, laundry, cleaning supplies, books and newspapers, clothes, etc.

4. A Swedish Reacher* will help the patient avoid bending to pick up objects.

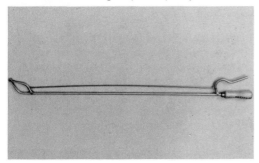

Swedish Reacher

Approach Toward Rehabilitation

Your approach and the patient's approach are very important in self-care training of the arthritic patient. You should not see the self-care training as merely a physical task on your part. The patient needs your constant support and reinforcement. Your encouragement of his independence and your praise for his efforts and successes, no matter how small, are extremely important. Emphasize the positive! Very disabled patients have proven that with positive attitude and motivation they can become independent with minimal adaptations.

Review: Answer the following questions.

1. *The maintenance of improper body position for a short period of time will result in stiffness, limited ROM, and, eventually, deformities. True or False*

2. *For a patient with trouble reaching his mouth as a result of restricted motion in the shoulder, which one of the following would you suggest?*
   a. *Built-up handle.*
   b. *Swivel spoon.*
   c. *Long-handled utensil.*
   d. *Utensil holder.*

3. *To gain strength, the patient should work until he is fatigued. True or False*

4. *For the arthritic patient, the easiest task of personal hygiene is combing his hair. True or False*

5. *Some of the hemiplegic procedures can be adapted for arthritics. True or False*

6. *The nurse told Mr. G. that dressing should be done in bed. True or False*

7. *Mrs. S. was told that she should eat lunch in bed since she has to have rest periods throughout the day. True or False*

8. *Mr. B. was pushing the armchair in his room, then he straightened up and held his back. It should not be the duty of the nurse who saw him to correct him. True or False*

Answers:

1. *True.*	3. *False.*	5. *True.*	7. *False.*
2. *c*	4. *False.*	6. *False.*	8. *False.*

Sources for Arthritis Information

The following references would be of great value to every disabled homemaker:

1. American Heart Association, 44 East 23rd Street, New York, New York 10010.
2. The Arthritis Foundation, 1212 Avenue of Americas, New York, New York 10036.
3. *Mealtime Manual for the Aged and Handicapped* prepared by the Institute of Rehabilitation Medicine, New York University Medical Center, Essandess Special Editions, a division of Simon and Schuster, Inc., 630 Fifth Avenue, New York, New York 10020. Available on order from bookstores or from Fashion-ABLE, spiral bound or paper on board.

Parkinsonism

Although you are probably familiar with Parkinsonism from Chapter 1 we shall review it again briefly. Parkinsonism, or the Parkinson's syndrome, is a chronic, slow progressing disease that is caused by damage to the basal ganglia in the brain. It is characterized

*J.A. Preston Corporation, 71 Fifth Avenue, New York, New York 10003.

by rigidity, tremor, and diminished automatic movements. Most cases are caused by an unknown factor. Others may be a result of post-encephalitis or an arteriosclerotic process. The typical clinical picture that the patient presents is loss of the facial expression, drooling saliva, slowing of functions, shuffling gait with no reciprocal movements, and trunk bent forward.

The three major disabling factors are:

1. *Rigidity.* Rigidity is caused by the increased muscle tone that is equally present in opposing muscle groups. There is muscle stiffness with resistance to both active and passive movements. The patient has trouble changing positions and in making starting and stopping movements.
2. *Tremor.* Tremors are involuntary movements which begin in one extremity and can gradually spread to the rest of the body and the head. The fingers and thumb move in characteristic motions called pill rolling movements. The tremor is present at rest, lessens during voluntary movements, and is absent at sleep.
3. *Lack of automatic movements.* There are no reciprocal motions, no blinking, and no expression on the face.

Review: Answer the following questions.

1. *Parkinsonism is characterized by joint stiffness, pain, and tremor. True or False*
2. *The tremor in Parkinsonism will increase with function. True or False*
3. *The Parkinson's patient will have no trouble getting up from a chair. True or False*
4. *Parkinsonism is a slow progressing, chronic disease. True or False*

Answers:

1. *False.*   3. *False.*
2. *False.*   4. *True.*

If your answers were correct proceed to the next section.

Self-Care Training

The completion of self-care activities by the patient helps him to maintain his coordination, ROM, endurance, the level at which he functions, and his morale. As a result, performing self-care activities daily is of the utmost importance. There are very few specific devices and procedures for self-care activities in Parkinsonism, therefore the emphasis should be on:

1. Establishing a routine in the patient's daily activities.
2. Letting the patient do as much as he possibly can without getting frustrated.
3. Keeping him interested in social activities.
4. Supporting his interests.
5. Encouraging him by praising his efforts (it usually takes awhile before you can praise any success).

When the patient's performance is very slow, remember that is part of his disease. You will find yourself wanting to do it for him, but *DON'T.* You should have plenty of patience and allow sufficient time to promote the patient's independece. Ultimately, this technique will raise the patient's self-esteem.

The self-help devices for the patient with Parkinsonism are used to help him perform his daily activities despite the tremor and rigidity and to assure the proper safety precautions. Weighted devices help to stabilize objects. Devices with extended handles help the patient reach the lower extremities.

Suggested rules in self-care training:

1. Instruct the patient to make one continuous motion. For example, in trying to drink the patient finds that after he picks up the cup he cannot reach it to his mouth due to the rigidity and tremor. He should put the cup down on the table, then pick it up and reach to his mouth in one continuous motion.
2. While instructing in self-care you might find it helpful to point out the destination of the movement to be performed, or quote the estimated distance. Instead of saying "Let's shave now," say "Let's shave now, pick up the razor;" you let him pick it up, and then you say, "Reach the razor to your cheek."
3. Use self-help devices only when necessary.
4. If the patient's endurance is low, use the following sequence of training: The patient starts by doing the easier task and graduates to the more difficult tasks.

5. Be patient. Let the patient feel your genuine interest in him and in his progress.

Review: Answer the following questions.

1. *Which of the following are characteristics of Parkinsonism?*
   a. *Joint disorders.*
   b. *Loss of sensation.*
   c. *Tremor.*
   d. *Rigidity.*
   e. *Paralysis.*
2. *Since the patient requires minimal assistance for his self-care but is very slow, the nurse, in order to be available for other duties, should go ahead and do it all for him. True or False*
3. *It is very important that the patient perform self-care activities and ADL daily to help maintain his endurance, ROM, and morale. True or False*

Answers:

1. *c, d*
2. *False.*
3. *True.*

If you answered all the questions correctly you are ready to proceed to the next section. Let us now look into the self-help devices used for Parkinson's patients.

Self-Help Devices for Eating

1. Use of unbreakable dishes is preferred.
2. A deep dish or a plate guard may be required.
3. If the plate has to be stabilized, use a suction cup or a wet washcloth placed underneath it.
4. If cutting the food is too difficult for the patient, it should be cut prior to serving.
5. For severe tremor, try a one pound wristlet placed on the forearm while the patient is eating. Use it for about a week and then see if the patient can perform the task without it. Do not use it if it does not help or annoys the patient.
6. For drinking, use of a weighted cup or a cup holder will prevent the cup from tipping over (see Arthritis section).

Personal Hygiene Procedures

The procedures for hemiplegics and arthritic patients can be applied to the Parkinsonism patient.

1. Use an electric razor for safety. Encourage the patient to move his head in all directions while shaving.
2. A wristlet might help for make-up procedures.
3. If the patient wears dentures and his coordination is poor, clean the dentures for him.
4. To avoid falls in the bath, the patient should be supervised, even if he is independent.

Dressing Procedures and Self-Help Devices

1. Recommended style of clothing:
   a. Wear clothes one size larger than usually worn.
   b. Wear clothes with roomy cuts.
   c. Use Velcro instead of buttons only if necessary. Buttoning and unbuttoning clothes is a good exercise (Velcro is available commercially).
   d. Have big buttons rather than small ones.
   e. On long sleeved shirts, adapt the regular buttons on cuffs by sewing a piece of elastic onto the button and keeping the cuffs buttoned, or by using Velcro or cufflinks.
   f. Attach a fabric tie or a metal ring to zippers.
2. To dress, the patient should be seated in an armchair. The procedures for the hemiplegic will probably be the easiest ones to apply. There is an additional procedure that is not recommended for one-handed patients or for arthritic patients but can be useful for the Parkinsonism patient when putting on or taking off shirts, sweaters, or coats that have front openings.
   a. Putting shirt on:
      (1) Put shirt on your knees, label facing down, collar toward the knees.

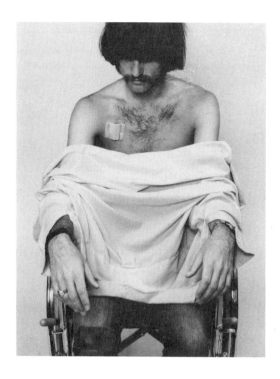

(2) Place your hands in the sleeves starting at the armhole. Reach through to the cuffs and push the shirt up over the elbows.

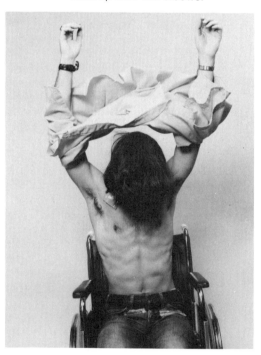

(3) Gather shirttail with both hands and pull shirt over head.
(4) Pull down on shirttail and straighten it up.
(5) Button.
b. Taking shirt off:
(1) Unbutton shirt and sleeves.
(2) Raise arms, bend elbows, place hands over shoulders.
(3) Gather shirt in back with both hands.
(4) Pull over head.
(5) Pull one sleeve off.
(6) Pull other sleeve off.
3. In putting on socks and shoes, the patient might require help in the beginning due to his stiffness. Shoes with buckles, elastic laces, or Velcro fasteners are preferable. The procedure for putting on socks and shoes can be done from crossed legs position or foot stool. Procedures can be adapted from the hemiplegic or the arthritic patient, depending on the patient's potential.

Activities of Daily Living

As discussed previously, ADL has a tremendous impact on the person's interest and happiness in life. The patient should be encouraged to visit other patients, read the paper, listen to the radio, keep up with his hobbies, and, if feasible, go and get the newspaper or write a letter. For writing practice the patient should start with large circles on large paper and continue with other prewriting exercises. As soon as this is managed, the same exercises should be done on lines one-half inch apart. The patient has to fill the entire space between the lines. The next stage will be writing in the space. You should make sure that the handwriting does not become smaller.

Review: Answer the following questions:

1. *A hemiplegic patient could use a stocking device. True or False*
2. *The Parkinsonism patient should put on a shirt the same way the arthritic patient does. True or False*
3. *A Parkinsonism patient could probably put on shoes the same way the arthritic and hemiplegic patients do. True or False*
4. *Mr. B., a Parkinsonism patient, welcomes*

you every morning with a big smile. *True or False*

5. The prewriting exercises for the Parkinsonism patient are necessary because of the rigidity and tremor. *True or False*

6. The benefits of performing self-care are not only independence or partial independence but improved endurance, ROM, and strength. *True or False*

Answers:

1. False.   4. False.
2. False.   5. True.
3. True.   6. True.

Posttest for Arthritis and Parkinsonism

Please circle the correct answer or answers for each item. When you are finished check your answers with those given.

1. The arthritic patient told you that he didn't do well at all today. Choose one statement as your reply:
   a. "It's going to take time before you realize how well you are doing."
   b. "You did as much as you could."
   c. "We all have good days and bad days."
   d. "I noticed that today you put on your blouse independently, yesterday you still required my assistance."

2. Mrs. B. has severe arthritis and she can't reach with the spoon to her mouth; you solved the problem by handing her a built-up spoon. *True or False*

3. You instructed Mr. S., an arthritic patient, in the use of a long-handled fork but he seemed uncooperative. You assumed that the reasons were:
   a. He didn't understand the instructions.
   b. He didn't want to use his hand since he was afraid of pain.
   c. He was afraid to fail.

4. The arthritic and Parkinson's patient should use an "Insert-A-Foot Shoe Aid" for putting on shoes. *True or False*

5. Mrs. K., an arthritic patient, is a very active person. Yesterday you saw her pick up her glasses by using incorrect body mechanics. What should you suggest?
   a. Bend her back and reach.

   b. Use a Swedish reacher.
   c. Bend her hips and knees and reach.

6. The major disabling factors in Parkinson's are:
   a. Pain.
   b. Perceptual problems.
   c. Intentional tremor.
   d. Rigidity.
   e. Diminished automatic movements.

7. The purpose of correct posture is to prevent pain. *True or False*

8. The self-help devices for the arthritic patient have to be lightweight. *True or False*

9. The Parkinsonism patient requires a lot of self-help devices. *True or False*

10. Mrs. G., a Parkinsonism patient, is very slow in her self-care activities. It's probably due to pain. *True or False*

11. Mrs. B. was admitted with the diagnosis of chronic rheumatoid arthritis for two weeks observation. Which of the following, regarding self-care, should the nurse do?
    a. Obtain information regarding the physical, mental, emotional, and social aspects.
    b. Knowing that the patient will stay for only a few days, not bother with training.
    c. Evaluate the patient's potential and set realistic goals.
    d. Ask the nurse's aide to help the patient as much as possible to make her comfortable and happy.

12. You, the nurse, are very busy but you should train the patient in self-care techniques to provide quality care and to promote the patient's maximal independence. *True or False*

13. Before purchasing expensive devices, you should try using self-help devices constructed by modifying existing articles. *True or False*

14. Arthritic patients will benefit from a weighted wristlet. *True or False*

15. An arthritic patient should put his socks on the same way a hemiplegic does. *True or False*

Answers:

1. d
2. False.
3. b and c.
4. False.

5. *If you answered b and c, you were correct. If a reacher is not available, c will be appropriate.*
6. *d and e.*
7. *False.*
8. *True.*
9. *False.*
10. *False.*
11. *a and c.*
12. *True.*
13. *True.*
14. *False.*
15. *False*

If you missed any of the posttest questions review the appropriate sections of this unit. Once you feel confident that you understand the material in this unit, please continue.

Suggestions for Establishing a Rehabilitation Program

The following practical suggestions based on clinical experience should serve as a useful guide as you plan a rehabilitation program in your own setting:

1. It would be beneficial for the patients and nursing staff to have a *room appropriated for meals and recreation.* The patients with adequate sitting endurance would have a chance to socialize, get out of their rooms, and get into a routine. This would also allow nurses to supervise larger numbers of patients. In addition, patients with an hour and a half sitting endurance can use this period for meals, since it is easier to eat when sitting up.

2. *Wearing street clothes* should be a routine in a rehabilitation center and a desired routine in a general hospital. Wearing clothes helps improve the patient's emotional condition, brings the patient back to a daily routine, and allows the patient to relearn to dress himself.

3. *Self-help devices* should be part of the supplies kept on the ward. Do not use them unless absolutely necessary, and keep them to a minimum. If a patient needs a device when discharged, he should be able to take it with him and the family should be instructed in its use.

4. Before attempting self-care training make sure that the *patient has passed the acute stage of his illness* and is medically ready for the effort of taking care of himself.

5. *Know the patient diagnosis, cause, and prognosis,* and if possible, know the patient's background before admission.

6. *Routine procedures have to be done daily,* the *same way,* and, when possible, at the same time. Staff members will need to be able to apply the different procedures and devices. Make sure that the staff members who treat the patient are consistent in their use of techniques and terminology and are aware of the patient's level of performance.

7. *Encourage the patient to do for himself as much as he can.* Praise every interest, effort, and success. Approach the goal of independence slowly and realistically. In the beginning you help as much as needed and your help will decrease with progress. Use the patient's potential, no matter how limited, until he reaches his maximal level of independence. Do not frustrate the patient by letting him fail or become overfatigued. Do not handle him unnecessarily.

8. Prior to training *explain to the patient:*
   a. what are you going to do,
   b. why you will do it,
   c. what you expect from him, and
   d. how he should help himself.

Do not ask him what he can do, i.e., "Can you eat by yourself?"

9. The best way to evaluate the patient's abilities and limitations will be to *determine,* through observation, *the level at which the patient functions* and the problems he faces.

10. The training plan and goals will *start from the level at which the patient functions,* and they will be broadened according to the patient's progress. Small training groups and repetitions have been found to be efficient and more stimulating to the patient.

11. *Informing staff and family on the patient's progress* and carry-over abilities avoids frustrations for everyone concerned.

Sources of Patient Aids

1. Be OK Self-Help Aids, Fred Sammons, Inc., P.O. Box 32, Brookfield, Illinois 60513.
2. Fashion-ABLE, Rocky Hill, New Jersey 08553.
3. Vocational Guidance of Rehabilitation Service, 2289 East 55th Street, Cleveland, Ohio 44103.

Catalogues are available on request.

Note

1. George L. Larsen, "Rehabilitation for Dysphagia Paralytica," *Journal of Speech and Hearing Disorders* 37 (May, 1972): 187-193.

Suggested Readings

Hirschberg, Lewis Thomas. *Rehabilitation — A Manual for the Care of the Disabled and Elderly.* Philadelphia: J. B. Lippincott, 1964.

Hollander, Joseph H. *Arthritis and Allied Conditions.* Philadelphia: Lea and Febiger, 1966.

Hurd, M. and Weylunis, G. W. "Shoulder Sling—Friend or Foe?" Archives of Physical Medicine and Rehabilitation 55 (1974), p. 519.

The Merck Manual of Diagnosis and Therapy. Rahway, N.J., and West Point. Pa.: Merck, Sharp and Dome Research Laboratories, Division of Merck and Company, Inc., 1966.

Rusk, Howard A., M.D. *Rehabilitation Medicine.* St. Louis: C. V. Mosby Company, 1971.

Stryker, Ruth Perin. *Rehabilitative Aspects of Acute and Chronic Nursing Care.* Philadelphia: W. B. Saunders Company, 1972.

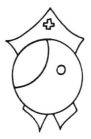

Wheelchairs:
Selection, Uses,
and Maintenance

Georgianna Wilson, L.P.T.
Virginia Kerr, O.T.R.

6.

Introduction and Objectives

Which wheelchair is best for your patient?

If you can solve this problem you can: help to enlarge your patient's world; add to his independence, safety, and comfort; and save him money. Although there are numerous types of wheelchairs and accessories, we shall confine our discussion to a manageable few.

Our basic objective for this chapter is to teach you to evaluate a given patient's wheelchair needs and select the appropriate wheelchair for him. Specifically, once you have completed this package you should be able to:

1. identify the basic parts of a wheelchair,
2. identify several wheelchair accessories and their uses,
3. properly measure a patient for a wheelchair,
4. identify proper procedures for maintaining a wheelchair,
5. adapt a given wheelchair to a particular patient problem, and
6. select the best wheelchair for a specific patient.

The Problem

Picture yourself on 2-West of Ole Bloomin' Springs Hospital. You are facing twelve patients with different wheelchair needs and twelve wheelchairs. You must get every patient out of bed. Your problem is to select the appropriate wheelchair for each patient. If you select the wrong wheelchair, various problems may arise, and some patients might not be able to get out of bed.

We shall begin by briefly describing each patient's condition and then the twelve wheelchairs available. Please read these descriptions and become familiar with them. Once you have done that, complete the instruction in this chapter. At the conclusion of the chapter you will be asked to select the proper wheelchair for each of the twelve patients.

These are the patients:

1. Mrs. H. has two long leg casts because of the arthritis in her knees. Her doctor is trying to straighten them out. She will be up in a wheelchair every day but will have to be lifted into it. She can walk a short distance with a walker.
2. Mrs. S. is a petite, 80-year-old lady. She weighs about 80 pounds and is very alert. She has some leg weakness and needs a wheelchair to get to the dining room.
3. Miss E. dove into a shallow lake and fractured her cervical spine at the C_4 level. She is now a quadriplegic and has been in bed for three months. This is her first time sitting.
4. Mrs. N. had anemia for two months. The doctors have it under control, but her legs are weak. She can get in and out of bed fairly well but tends to get confused and gets her feet tangled. This makes her stumble. She walks short distances with a walker.
5. Mrs. R. has breast cancer. She had surgery seven days ago and now has physical therapy treatments to loosen her arm. She has to go to the third floor for her treatments.
6. Mrs. A. had a cerebrovascular accident three weeks ago. She is five feet tall. She wants to wheel her own wheelchair. She

has no movement in her left arm or leg. She has a very large stomach and cannot wiggle very well.
7. Mr. W. is 11 years old and has a fractured left ankle. He was jumping a ditch full of water and twisted his ankle when he landed. He had to have surgery to correct the break.
8. Mrs. B. has had a total hip replacement. She cannot flex her hip beyond 45°. She has been walking with a walker.
9. Mr. L. is five feet nine inches and has a left hemiplegia. He wheels his wheelchair using one arm and one leg. He has hemianopsia, poor sitting balance, and poor head control.
10. Mr. G. is 20. He fell off a telephone pole while at work and broke his back at L_2 and L_3. He is a paraplegic. He transfers independently by sliding from the bed to a wheelchair. He will be going back to school.
11. Mrs. O. fell over a cat at home and fractured her left hip. Since her hip surgery, she can only bend her knee to a 60° angle without a lot of pain. She weighs at least 250 pounds and loves to eat.
12. Mr. U. has a left hemiplegia and his leg swells. He is wearing an elastic stocking to decrease swelling. He stands up well and walks using a cane with minimal assistance.

These are the wheelchairs available:

1. Hemi wheelchair with removable legs and brake extension.
2. Full reclining wheelchair with elevating legs, removable arms, and head rest.
3. Semi-reclining wheelchair with elevating legs and removable arms.
4. Standard adult wheelchair with elevating removable legs.
5. Standard adult chair with hook-on head rest, toggle brakes, and hard roll insert.
6. Standard adult wheelchair with swinging detachable leg rests.
7. Standard adult wheelchair with removable desk arms, regular removable legs, heel loops, pneumatic tires.
8. Standard wheelchair with removable arms and removable elevating leg rests.
9. Narrow adult chair with removable legs.

10. Extra wide adult chair with elevating legs, removable arms, and brake lever extensions.
11. Junior wheelchair with elevating legs.
12. Standard adult chair with lever brakes.

The information you need to identify the appropriate chair for each patient is contained in the following pages.

The Standard Wheelchair

Standard model wheelchairs incorporate the wheelchair dimensions used most frequently by patients. The most commonly used standard models include, the *adult, narrow adult,* and *junior chair.*

The standard dimensions need not be memorized since they are located in all wheelchair catalogs and manuals. When checking the measurements, be sure to note the overall width of the chair to determine if it will clear doorways. Also note that the wheelchair's turning radius is four and a half feet when maneuvered expertly and more when less expertly maneuvered (see Table 6-1).

Some wheelchairs with the dimensions given below are available in a lighter weight. Have you ever tried wrestling a wheelchair into a car? Sometimes this is quite a chore. Picture yourself as the elderly wife of a patient or as a partially disabled patient engaged in this struggle. Lightweight chairs are fifty percent lighter than standard chairs. They are a little less durable, but they are much easier to handle.

Wheelchair Parts

Correct identification of wheelchair features and components is essential when you wish to select a wheelchair. (See Figure 6-1.) The right and left sides are determined by sitting in the chair.

1. Arm
2. Arm Rest
3. Back
4. Seat
5. Skirt Guard
6. Foot Rest
7. Foot Plate
8. Brake
9. Wheel
10. Hand Rim
11. Caster
12. Hand Grip
13. Tipping Lever

TABLE 6-1
Standard Wheelchair Dimensions*

	Adult	Narrow Adult	Junior
Width of seat at seat level	18"	16"	16"
Width overall—open	26"	23"	23"
Width overall—closed	10"	10"	10"
Seat depth	16"	16"	14"
Back height	16"	16"	16"
Arm to seat	10"	10"	9"
Seat to floor	20"	20"	18"
Overall length	42"	42"	39"
Overall height	37"	37"	37"
Seat to foot rest—minimum	15"	15"	13"
Seat to foot rest—maximum	20"	20"	17"
Net weight	47 lbs.	45 lbs.	45 lbs.

* All dimensions are to the nearest inch.

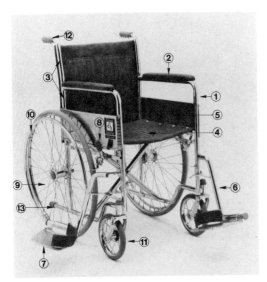

Figure 6-1

Study the wheelchair components as identified, then cover the numbered list of components, and fill in the blanks with the correct numbers.

____ Arm   ____ Foot Plate
____ Wheel   ____ Foot Rest
____ Tipping Lever   ____ Caster
____ Hand Rim   ____ Brake
____ Hand Grip   ____ Back
____ Skirt Guard   ____ Arm Rest
                 ____ Seat

If your numbers and components match up as follows, you have done well for the first time. If they do not match, study the diagram more carefully before you proceed.

1	Arm	6	Foot Rest
9	Wheel	11	Caster
13	Tipping Lever	8	Brake
10	Hand Rim	3	Back
12	Hand Grip	2	Arm Rest
5	Skirt Guard	4	Seat
7	Foot Plate		

Function and Adaptation of Wheelchair Parts

Now that you know the names of the wheelchair parts, you need to know their functions and what you can do to adapt a given part to a particular patient problem.

Wheelchair Arms

There are three types of arms available:

1. Standard arms, as pictured in Figure 6-1, come with most chairs.

2. Desk arms are shortened to allow the chair to fit under a desk, table, etc.

3. Detachable arms can be removed by pressing a release button. They are necessary when a patient cannot stand up to perform a standing transfer and must slide from the wheelchair to his bed. (See Chapter 2 for Transfers.) Patients requiring detachable arms are paraplegics, those with long leg casts, or those with limited ROM at the knees or hips. Detachable arms are also desirable when transferring a total care patient because you do not have to lift him over the wheelchair arms.

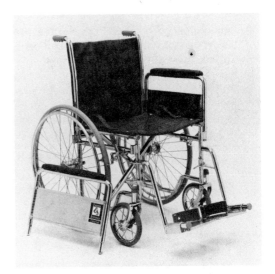

Wheelchair arm height is measured from the wheelchair seat to the patient's bent elbow plus one inch. Remember, if you use a seat cushion, its height should be considered when measuring for correct arm height. Thus, standard arm height is important if the patient will be confined to the wheelchair for life. Then the proper height not only adds comfort but helps to prevent deformities and aids the patient in doing adequate wheelchair pushups. (See illustration on next page.)

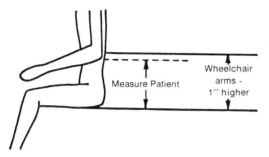

Measure Patient

Wheelchair arms - 1″ higher

Refer back to pg. 163 for your list of patients. For which of your patients should you be concerned about wheelchair arm height?

Answer _____

If you answered *Miss E., patient no. 3,* you are correct.

Wheelchair Back

Four wheelchair backs are available:

1. Standard is the straight back pictured in Figure 6-1.
2. Semireclining reclines from vertical to 30°. A patient with a hip prosthesis cannot flex past 45° and would require this type or a full reclining back.
3. Full reclining backs or Neurochairs recline to the horizontal. They are used to reduce frequency of patient transfers, or to slowly increase a patient's tolerance to sitting erect.

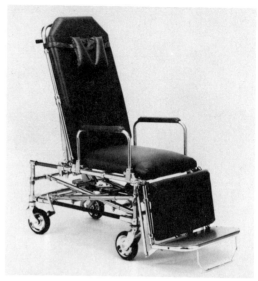

Neurochairs

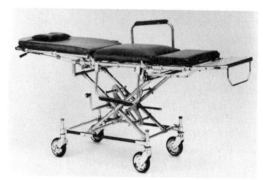

Horizontal Recline

4. Hook-on head rests can go on any of the above to support the head of a very weak patient or one with very poor head control. If a head rest is not available use a padded back board that extends to head level.

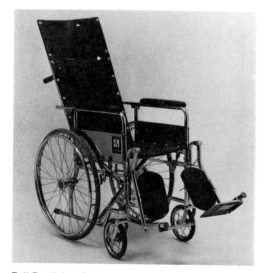

Full Reclining Backs

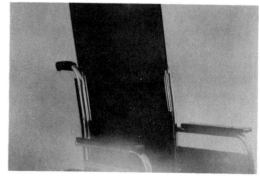

Which of your assigned patients needs the extra head support provided by a hook-on head rest? Answer _____

If you wrote *Mr. L., patient no. 9,* you are correct.

Proper back height helps to maintain proper posture and trunk support. But, again, standard back height will do in most cases.

1. A patient requiring full trunk support would need a semi- or full reclining back.
2. For minimal trunk support the wheelchair back should come to approximately four inches below the patient's armpit.

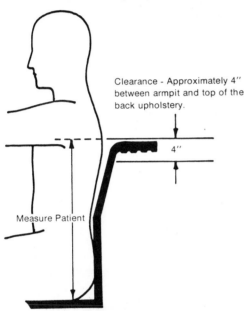

Clearance - Approximately 4" between armpit and top of the back upholstery.

4"

Measure Patient

Wheelchair Skirt Guards

Skirt Guards are the side panels attached to the wheelchair arms. They prevent a patient's clothes from becoming entangled in the wheels.

Wheelchair Seat

A standard sling seat as pictured in Figure 6-1 is satisfactory for most patients. *Note:* Be sure the upholstery is urine proof— naugahyde and not canvas.

Measurements are taken as follows:

1. Seat width is measured from the sides of skirtguards and is approximately two inches wider than the patient. Keep the seat width as narrow as possible to reduce the overall width of the wheelchair. (Standard Adult = 18" seat width; Narrow Adult = 16" seat width; Junior = 16" seat width.) Which of your assigned patients could use a Narrow Adult chair?

Answer: _____

If you wrote *Mrs. S., patient no. 2,* you are correct.

2. Seat depth should be approximately two to three inches less than the patient's thigh measurement. Just remember that you should be able to place three or four fingers between the rear of the patient's knee and the edge of the seat.

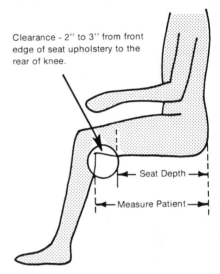

Clearance - 2" to 3" from front edge of seat upholstery to the rear of knee.

Seat Depth

Measure Patient

3. A hemi chair seat is of standard width, but it is set lower to the floor. This enables the short hemiplegic patient to touch the floor with his uninvolved leg and propel his chair (see Chapter 2 on Wheelchair Ambulation).

Adaptations—There are different types and sizes of *cushions* that aid comfort and help prevent pressure sores. Cushions also allow the patient to stand up more easily. However, if the cushion is too thick, your hemiplegic patient may not be able to touch the floor and will thus be unable to manipulate his wheelchair.

Hard rolls can be rolled up bed pads and can be used to aid a hemiplegic patient with very poor sitting balance who continually leans to his affected side. You may be accustomed to seeing such patients propped up with pillows stuffed between them and the wheelchair on their affected side. *Instead* place the hard roll you made between the patient's hips and the skirt guard on his *unaffected side*. This prevents him from moving his hips up against the skirt guard and prevents him from leaning so far to one side.

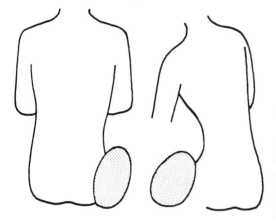

Which of your patients needs a hard roll?

Answer _____

If you wrote *Mr. L., patient no. 9*, you are correct.

A solid insert to act as a *seat board* can be purchased or made from any padded board to assist the patient in maintaining a proper sitting position. Remember that this changes the seat height just as cushions do. A cut out seat board with a cushion on top may be used to help prevent pressure sores. (See also Chapter 9.)

Wheelchair Foot Rests

Foot Rests come in three types:

1. Standard foot rests are attached to the chair as shown in Figure 6-1.
2. Swinging, detachable foot rests lock into place or swing to the side by releasing a button. They can also be removed for close approaches to bed or tub and to allow easy loading into cars.
3. Swinging, detachable, elevating leg rests are recommended as an aid in lower extremity circulation or any lower extremity injury where edema is present.

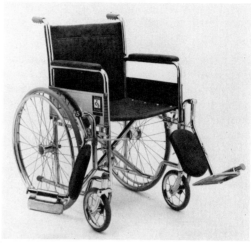

Measure the patient from the rear of the bent knee to the heel of the foot. All foot rests are adjustable and should be adjusted properly for comfort and proper weight distribution on the thighs and buttocks. The patient's thigh must be elevated slightly (approximately two fingers width) above the front edge of the seat upholstery. Also the lowest point of the foot plate should clear the floor by at least two inches.

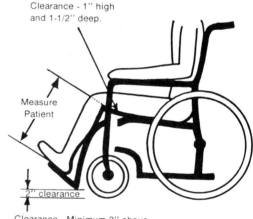

Clearance - 1" high and 1-1/2" deep.

Measure Patient

2" clearance

Clearance - Minimum 2" above floor for safety.

Some foot rests have a bolt on the bottom of the foot plate and some have it on the side. To adjust the foot rests, have the patient sit in the wheelchair with his feet in the middle of the foot plates. Loosen the bolt and push in or pull out on the foot plate to achieve the correct height. Tighten the bolt. Learn how to do this. It is not difficult to do and makes a big difference in patient comfort.

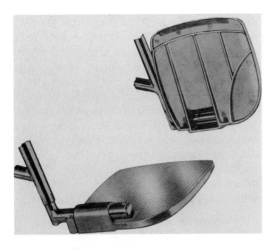

Wheelchair Foot Plates

Standard *foot plates* flip up for safe exit from the chair. *Heel loops* help to hold flailing legs in place. This is especially helpful on wheelchairs with elevating leg rests. *Toe loops* help hold spastic legs in place.

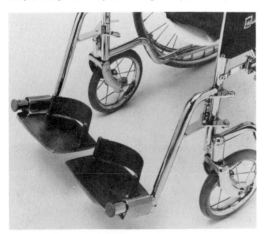

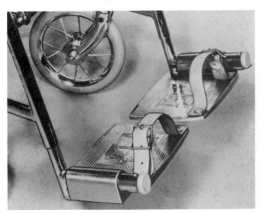

Safety note: Be careful that the foot plates are up and that they stay up before allowing a patient to exit a wheelchair.

Wheelchair Brakes

Standard *toggle brakes* are the safest and easiest to operate. Push-type locking action brakes are standard; however, pull action are available. *Lever brakes* have separate locking latches. These are easily bent out of shape, so they do not always lock securely. Also, elderly, confused patients or those with perceptual problems might not always get them into the last notch. For these reasons, lever brakes are not recommended. *Brake lever extensions* can be added to give better leverage. They require less strength and are helpful when you have a very weak patient or one with limited range of motion. They are also useful for hemiplegics who cannot reach over to the brake or who cannot find it. However, not all hemiplegics require them.

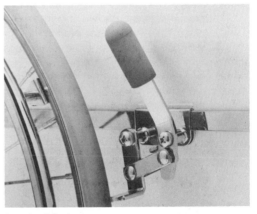

Standard Brakes

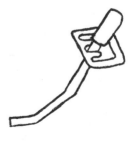

Lever Brakes

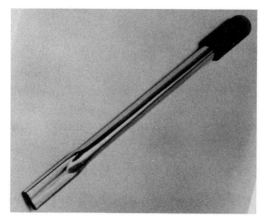

Brake Extensions

Which one of your assigned patients could use a brake extension?

Answer _____

If you answered *Mrs. O., patient no. 11,* or *Mrs. A., patient no. 6,* you are correct.

Wheelchair Wheels

Standard wheels are shown in Figure 6-1. They are 24 inches in diameter. Notice that the wheel and hand rim are separate pieces. Lightweight wheels have the wheel and hand rim as one piece. Solid rubber tires are standard, but pneumatic tires of 1 3/4 inches or 1 1/4 inches width are recommended for patients who will be using their wheelchairs outside on grass, sand, or uneven surfaces. You should consider your patient's occupation before ordering tires. *Spoke guards* can be ordered on wheelchairs, or they

can be made by cutting a circle from plastic or cardboard and taping it to the spokes. These are helpful with patients who have flailing arms or arms with poor sensation that might become caught in the wheel spokes and injured.

Standard *handrims*, as shown in Figure 6-1, are chrome plated. There are rubber covers that slip on to improve friction; plastic coating also provides greater friction. Special handrims are available for patients who have difficulty grasping, such as quadriplegics, arthritics, etc. Handrims can be pushed with:

1. rubber tipped horizontal projections,
2. rubber tipped oblique projections, or
3. rubber tipped vertical projections.

The patient can push against the projections with the heel of his hand. *Note:* Special purpose handrims can be used depending upon the patient's needs—either chrome plated or plastic coated. They are recommended when an individual has difficulty in grasping regular handrims.

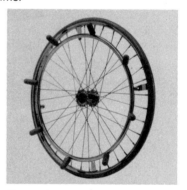

Rubber Tipped Oblique Projections

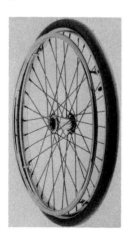
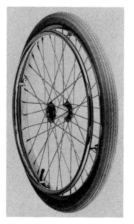

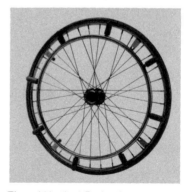

Rubber Tipped Vertical Projections

Standard *caster wheels* are eight inches in diameter and are hard rubber, as shown on p. 165. They come with the different tires discussed above.

Wheelchair Tipping Lever

Tipping levers are the horizontal projections at the bottom and back of the wheelchair. By placing your foot on one of them and pulling back on the hand grips you can tip the front of the wheelchair up off the ground to move it over a door facing, electric cord, curb, etc. Never try to just push the chair over an obstacle—the caster can get caught and throw the patient out of the chair.

Now for your big project. . .

Posttest

Directions: Repeated here is a list of the patients that have been assigned to you and the wheelchairs that are available to sit them in. Select the proper wheelchair for each patient (use the answer sheet, pg. 172) and then check your answers, pg. 172. Are you going to be able to get all of your patients out of bed?

These are the patients:

1. *Mrs. H. has two long leg casts because of the arthritis in her knees. The doctor is trying to straighten them out. She will be up in a wheelchair every day but will have to be lifted into it. She can walk a short distance with a walker.*
2. *Mrs. S. is a petite, 80-year-old lady. She weighs about 80 pounds and is very alert. She has some leg weakness and needs a wheelchair to get to the dining room.*
3. *Miss E. dove into a shallow lake and fractured her cervical spine at C_4. She is now a quadriplegic and has been in bed for three months. This is her first time sitting.*
4. *Mrs. N. had anemia for two months. The doctors have it under control, but her legs are weak. She can get in and out of bed fairly well but tends to become confused and get her feet tangled. This makes her stumble. She walks short distances with a walker.*

5. *Mrs. R. has breast cancer. She had surgery seven days ago and now has physical therapy treatments to loosen her arm. She has to go to the third floor for her treatments.*
6. *Mrs. A. had a cerebrovascular accident three weeks ago. She is five feet tall. She wants to wheel her own wheelchair. She has no movement in her left arm or leg. She has a very large stomach and cannot wiggle very well.*
7. *Mr. W. is 11 years old and has a fractured left ankle. He was jumping a ditch full of water and twisted his ankle when he landed. He had to have surgery to correct the break.*
8. *Mrs. B. has had a total hip replacement. She cannot flex her hip beyond 45°. She has been walking with a walker.*
9. *Mr. L. is five feet nine inches and has a left hemiplegia. He wheels his wheelchair using one arm and one leg. He has hemianopsia, poor sitting balance, and poor head control.*
10. *Mr. G. is 20. He fell off a telephone pole while at work and broke his back at L_2 and L_3. He is a paraplegic. He transfers independently by sliding from the bed to a wheelchair. He will be going back to school.*
11. *Mrs. O. fell over a cat at home and fractured her left hip. Since her hip surgery she can only bend her knee to a 60° angle without a lot of pain. She weighs at least 250 pounds and loves to eat.*
12. *Mr. U. has a left hemiplegia and his leg swells. He is wearing an elastic stocking to decrease swelling. He stands up well and walks using a cane with minimal assistance.*

These are the wheelchairs which are available:

1. *Hemi wheelchair with removable legs and brake extension.*
2. *Full reclining wheelchair with elevating legs, removable arms, and head rest.*
3. *Semi reclining wheelchair with elevating legs and removable arms.*
4. *Standard adult wheelchair with elevating removable legs.*
5. *Standard adult chair with hook-on head*

rest, toggle brakes, and hard roll insert.

6. Standard adult wheelchair with swinging detachable leg rests.
7. Standard adult wheelchair with removable desk arms, regular removable legs, heel loops, pneumatic tires.
8. Standard wheelchair with removable arms and removable elevating leg rests.
9. Narrow adult chair with removable legs.
10. Extra wide adult chair with elevating legs, removable arms, and brake lever extensions.
11. Junior wheelchair with elevating legs.
12. Standard adult chair with lever brakes.

ANSWER SHEET

Directions: Mark the appropriate patient's name and number on the line available, i.e., wheelchair No. 30 should be fitted to Mr. Z., patient No. 20.

PATIENT NAME   NUMBER

Wheelchair No. 1   _____
Wheelchair No. 2   _____
Wheelchair No. 3   _____
Wheelchair No. 4   _____
Wheelchair No. 5   _____
Wheelchair No. 6   _____
Wheelchair No. 7   _____
Wheelchair No. 8   _____
Wheelchair No. 9   _____
Wheelchair No. 10   _____
Wheelchair No. 11   _____
Wheelchair No. 12   _____

When you are finished, check your answers with those given below.

Answers:

Wheelchair No. 1:   Mrs. A., Patient No. 6
Wheelchair No. 2:   Miss E., Patient No. 3
Wheelchair No. 3:   Mrs. B., Patient No. 8
Wheelchair No. 4:   Mr. U., Patient No. 12
Wheelchair No. 5:   Mr. L., Patient No. 9
Wheelchair No. 6:   Mrs. N., Patient No. 4
Wheelchair No. 7:   Mr. G., Patient No. 10
Wheelchair No. 8:   Mrs. H, Patient No. 1
Wheelchair No. 9:   Mrs. S., Patient No. 2
Wheelchair No. 10:   Mrs. O., Patient No. 11
Wheelchair No. 11:   Mr. W., Patient No. 7
Wheelchair No. 12:   Mrs. R., Patient No. 5

If you answered correctly, each of your patients will have the proper chair. If you did not, some of your patients will still be in bed! If they are "still in bed," rework the list and use the chapter as a reference. In a real life situation it is very important to switch wheelchairs until the proper chair is obtained for your patient.

Wheelchair Maintenance

We have just discussed the most important aspect of wheelchairs, that is, matching the patient with the correct chair. But for that chair to continue to be good for that particular patient, it must be properly maintained. Basic maintenance involves keeping the chair clean, dry, protected from the weather, and repaired when needed.

To clean your wheelchair, use a mild soap and water solution and be sure to wipe dry. Never use an abrasive on the chrome, and pay special attention to the wheels and casters to keep them free of lint, string, hair, and dirt. Rub the telescoping parts with paraffin to prevent sticking. Do not use oil on these parts because it collects dirt.

Never force a wheelchair to open or close. To close most wheelchairs, pull up on the seat by placing your hands on the front and the back of the upholstery. Some wheelchairs have upholstery handles provided on the sides of the seats; to close these, pull up on the handles. To open, push *down* on the sides of the seat. Never push *out* on the arms of the chair. This can "spring" the frame of the chair.

These simple measures plus a yearly checkup by a reputable wheelchair dealer can help prevent costly repairs. Also never force the car trunk lid down on a wheelchair.

Conclusion

Which wheelchair is best for your patient?

Now you know. In this chapter we have established a hypothetical, ideal situation for proper wheelchair selection. We know that you will not always have all of these types of wheelchairs available. Do not hesitate to adapt the chairs you do have to fit your patients. Some modifications can be made by simply adding cushions or adjusting foot rests. Be critical about accessories. Before acquiring accessories, be certain that the patient needs them either temporarily or for long term use. They do increase the cost of a wheelchair, and, in some instances, they make a wheelchair cumbersome and require extra maintenance. Our simple advice to you is— use the simplest wheelchair possible to fit your patient's needs.

Suggested Readings

Buchwald, E.; Rusk, H. A.; Deaver, G. G.; and Covalt, D. A. *Physical Rehabilitation for Daily Living.* New York: McGraw Hill, 1952.

Everest & Jennings, Inc. *Wheelchair Features and Benefits.* Los Angeles: Everest & Jennings, 1968.

Everest & Jennings, Inc. *Wheelchair Prescription—Measuring the Patient.* Los Angeles: Everest & Jennings, 1968.

Stryker, Ruth. *Rehabilitative Aspects of Acute and Chronic Nursing Care.* Philadelphia: W. B. Saunders Co., 1972.

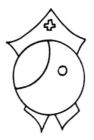

Identification and Management of Bowel Problems

ROBERT D. SINE, M.D.

7.

Introduction and Objectives

The identification and management of bowel problems are very important aspects of the management of rehabilitation patients. Here, we attempt to give insight into the nature of the problem and its alleviation and to offer helpful suggestions pertaining to the establishment of bowel control. Once you have completed this chapter you should be able to:

1. Differentiate between normal and abnormal bowel habits.
2. Identify causes for the interruption of normal bowel habits.
3. Recognize proper management procedures to handle specific bowel problems pertaining to constipation, diarrhea, and the neurogenic bowel.
4. Recognize the role that diet, fluids, physical activity, and timing play in formulating habit training for bowel control.
5. Identify a procedure that could be followed when planning a specific patient's bowel training program.

Pathophysiology

The two conditions that confront us most commonly are diarrhea and constipation. Both are produced by stool spending an abnormal duration in the colon. The ability of the colon to extract water from the stool accounts for the change from the watery stool entering it to the well-formed stool found in the rectum.

Diarrhea occurs when an irritable bowel with increased peristalsis hurries the stool, shortening the time available for water resorption. The resulting stools are frequent and watery. Any irritating agent can initiate the process. Most commonly, that agent is infectious; but toxic agents, especially drug side effects, are prevalant in hospital populations.

Decreasing peristalsis has the opposite effect, prolonging the duration of the stool within the colon and causing excess water extraction. Infrequent, hard stools (constipation) result. The process tends to perpetuate itself: the stool is hard to pass and slows the passage of that behind it, which, in turn, hardens. Stool continues to harden and accumulate until the condition is relieved.

Prophylaxis

Among the many causes of constipation, probably the most prevalent in a hospital population is inactivity, especially among bed rest patients. Inadequate dietary bulk and/or water intake are other very common offenders in the general population. Prophylaxis requires particular attention to these three factors. In patients who cannot be taken off bed rest or given adequate dietary bulk, stool softeners given prophylactically can be helpful.

Diagnosis

Now everybody knows how to diagnose constipation and diarrhea, right? No. You would do well to take the proverbial nickel for every gastro-intestinal series done because of these syndromes.

Small infrequent evacuations of hard stool are the hallmarks of constipation. As the condition advances cramps, distension, anorexia, and even elevation of white count and temperature can appear. Palpation of the abdomen may show tenderness in the left lower quadrant in early cases. In late cases tenderness is more diffuse and an unmistakable "doughy" feel can be present. The finger can leave an impression if pressed forcefully into the abdomen as if pressing into clay.

The most frequent cause of confusion in making an early, correct diagnosis, particularly in the geriatric group, is when watery stools leak around an impaction, creating a condition that simulates diarrhea. This calls for disimpaction and treatment of the constipation. Treating for diarrhea can, of course, aggravate the situation a great deal. You can also be led astray by an evacuation that represents only a small part of a large accumulation of feces. None of these errors will occur if you will properly evaluate and include palpation of the abdomen in your evaluation.

A flat plate of the abdomen is helpful in doubtful cases. Digital examination is also helpful as there normally should not be feces in the rectum.

Treatment

We feel that "laxative of choice" usually turns out to be whatever "worked" last and is a hit or miss method of treating a very troublesome and potentially chronic problem. Any therapy should begin with evaluation of the severity of the condition, and constipation is no exception. Overtreatment is worse yet, as incontinence or diarrhea can result, which is then itself overtreated. The patient can be chronically whip-sawed between constipation and diarrhea.

Evaluation for treatment can be made by estimating the degree of accumulation of colonic contents (see Table 7-1). The top three boxes are stages of progressive accumulation. You begin by determining within which group your patient falls using the findings mentioned. The next tier of boxes suggests treatment appropriate for the condition. Many of the common laxatives work by drawing large amounts of water into the colon, which increases the volume within it and causes reflex peristalsis (Metamucil, MOM). They can be used on a sluggish, nondistended colon. Obviously this is not a reasonable approach (although it might work) in the face of an already distended colon. Drugs that act primarily on the colon's neural plexus without causing irritation of the wall—Senna (Senacott) and bisocodyl (Dulcolax)—are indicated. If the primary therapy is not effective you should not hesitate to move to reevaluation (the third tier of boxes) and further therapy. Again, the choice of enema, if indicated, should be appropriate to the findings on evaluation.

No drug, oral or rectal, should be repeated without digital examination. If impaction is present, the use of laxative forces the colon to attempt to move feces with nowhere to go. Cramps result. The longer the exam is avoided, the harder the impaction and the larger the accumulation. Once disimpaction is accomplished, enemas can be used freely and are effective. Oil is helpful when stool is hard,

TABLE 7-1
Management of Constipation

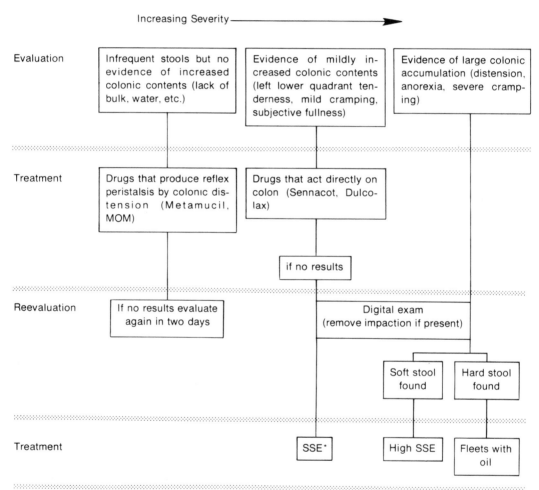

Increasing Severity ⟶

| Evaluation | Infrequent stools but no evidence of increased colonic contents (lack of bulk, water, etc.) | Evidence of mildly increased colonic contents (left lower quadrant tenderness, mild cramping, subjective fullness) | Evidence of large colonic accumulation (distension, anorexia, severe cramping) |

Treatment — Drugs that produce reflex peristalsis by colonic distension (Metamucil, MOM) — Drugs that act directly on colon (Sennacot, Dulcolax)

if no results

Reevaluation — If no results evaluate again in two days — Digital exam (remove impaction if present)

Soft stool found — Hard stool found

Treatment — SSE* — High SSE — Fleets with oil

Prophylaxis — Maintain bulk and water intake. Initiate stool softener until texture satisfactory. Mobilize if possible—use commode. Establish routine for defecation—avoid bed pan.

*Soap suds enema

and high enemas might be required when accumulations are large.

Finally, each episode should call attention to the importance of prophylaxis.

Neurogenic Bowel

The neurogenic bowel is a special case in bowel management. Peristalsis, which is retained in the spinal cord patient, is under autonomic nervous system control. It is generally sluggish, however, so the patient is vulnerable to constipation. Additionally, he does not feel the rectum fill and cannot "answer the call" by using the commode at the appropriate time, exerting control of his anal sphincters, or using his abdominal muscles to "bear down." Incontinence might be a problem as well. This symptom alone can be enough of a social nemesis to produce a shut-in.

While bowel management is often termed "bowel training," it is well to remember the common clinical warning "you don't train the bowel—it trains you." In practical terms, this means any "routine" must be the bowel's routine—not ours. If you are flexible you can bend it enough to fit into a daily schedule, but attempts to overregulate could result in the spinal cord patient's dread—incontinence at work or play.

The previous section's remarks for constipation prophylaxis should be reviewed and are even more important in the face of a neurogenic bowel. We routinely add stool softeners, but these should be discontinued if stools become watery.

Attempts to initiate evacuation should follow a hot meal with tea or coffee by about one-half hour. The patient should be comfortably seated on a commode. A large glycerin suppository can be used to initiate reflex evacuation. If this is not successful, digital massage and distension of the anal sphincter can be attempted—by the patient, if at all possible. If there is still no evacuation, attempts should be dropped until the following day. Medication, chosen according to the criteria in the prior section, can be used eight hours before the next attempt. The second day the procedure is repeated. A Dulcolax suppository can be added.

Enemas are to be avoided if at all possible!

Impactions are common, and huge accumulations of stool can occur painlessly. Digital exam should follow any suspicion of a problem. Keeping a good record can be crucial.

Summary

To initiate an evacuation provide or do the following:

1. A hot meal with tea or coffee.
2. One-half hour later, comfortable seating on commode.
3. If no evacuation, large glycerin suppository.
4. If no evacuation, massage of anal sphincter.
5. If no evacuation, medication eight hours prior to next attempt.
6. Repeat steps 1 through 4.
7. If no results, Dulcolax suppository.

Maintenance activities include:

1. Maintain a soft stool: adequate bulk, water, and stool softeners.
2. Check frequently for impaction.
3. Check abdomen frequently for stool accumulation.
4. Avoid enemas.
5. Avoid overtreating—a state of mild constipation is preferable to episodes of incontinence.

A spinal cord patient will not die of an unmanaged bowel. The complications of constipation and incontinence, however, can result in episodic illness and paralyzing social fears. Social and vocational horizons can constrict to within the tight radius of the commode—all for want of personnel with some skill and lots of patience.

Now let's see how much you have learned. Select the correct answers to the following.

Posttest

1. A hyperactive colon:
   a. can lead to constipation.
   b. prolongs the duration stool spends within the colon.
   c. results in hard, dry, stools.
   d. may be a drug side effect.
   e. all the above.
2. Prophylaxis in bowel management does not include:
   a. maintaining physical activity.
   b. maintaining water intake.
   c. daily use of a gentle laxative.
   d. maintaining dietary bulk.
3. Symptoms of constipation do not include:
   a. myalgia.
   b. cramps.
   c. anorexia.
   d. elevated temperature and white count.
   e. distension.
4. In a patient with constipation, cramping, and tenderness, and in which Senna has not resulted in evacuation, the next step is:
   a. high soap suds enema.
   b. Metamucil.
   c. digital exam.
   d. Fleet enema with oil.
5. The patient with neurogenic bowel retains:
   a. anal sphincter control.
   b. peristalsis.
   c. sensation of rectal filling.
   d. ability to "bear down."
6. In managing the neurogenic bowel there is no need to:
   a. observe frequently for distension.
   b. produce an evacuation every second day by enema.
   c. check digitally if there is suspicion of impaction.
   d. maintain a soft stool using stool softener if necessary.
   e. avoid incontinence allowing mild constipation if necessary.

Answers:

1. d	4. c
2. c	5. b
3. a	6. b

If you missed any of the posttest, you should review that section of this chapter.

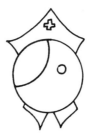

Identification and Management of Bladder Problems

Shelly E. Liss, M.D.

8.

Introduction and Objectives

The goal of bladder training is to achieve filling and emptying of the bladder as normally as possible for the individual patient. Mrs. Geriatric will be our patient for this lesson. We will begin by reviewing her physiological problem, why she has a problem, and what her incontinence implies.

Upon completion of this learning experience you will be able to:

1. Identify normal physiology and anatomy of the urinary tract.
2. Identify four types of incontinence.
3. Describe proper catheter care.
4. Identify complications of incontinence.
5. Identify pertinent questions and information to be gathered from the patient and family before devising a care plan.
6. Identify factors involved in bladder control and training.
7. Formulate a bladder training program and care plan, using knowledge gained in this chapter.

Figure 8-1 provides an outline for the male and female urinary systems. Please review this outline to refresh your memory of this portion of human anatomy.

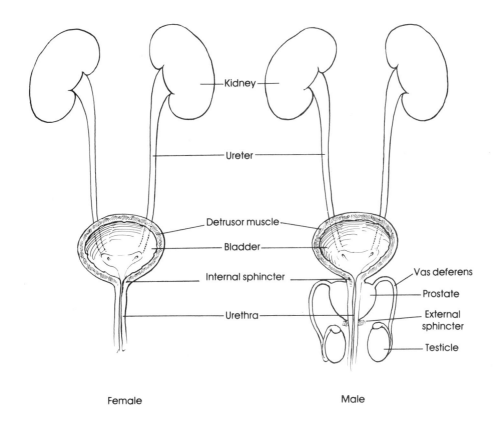

Figure 8-1 Identification and Management of Bladder Problems

Voiding

Urine enters the bladder, producing tension in the bladder wall to threshold level, causing the detrusor muscle fibers to stretch. Sensory impulses resulting from bladder pressure go to the central nervous system, and motor impulses return to the bladder. These return impulses produce detrusor muscle contraction waves; the external sphincter relaxes and voiding occurs. (Cerebral control can cause both voluntary inhibition of reflex, as well as voluntary initiation.)

Types of Incontinence

1. *Stress Incontinence.* This is most commonly seen in females with relaxation of pelvic musculature secondary to child birth. The patient loses urine when she coughs, sneezes, or strains. She does not feel the need to void but the urethral pressure is incapable of holding back the urine.

2. *Urge Incontinence.* This is the most common type of incontinence in the elderly. This can be secondary to bladder irritation, from infection, or caused by the patient's inability to inhibit the urge to void because of brain damage, as in senility or a stroke. These patients feel the urge to void. Proper antibiotics are required to treat the infection. Bladder training should be tried in the brain damaged.

3. *Incontinence of High Spinal Cord Dysfunction.* This is seen in "high" paraplegics and quadriplegics. The bladder

empties without the patient feeling the urge to void or being able to inhibit voiding. The bladder is working through the spinal reflex, which has been disconnected from the brain. These patients can learn to initiate the reflex by stroking their abdomen or some other trigger mechanism if the pelvic musculature is not too spastic to allow the bladder to empty.

4. *Incontinence of Low Spinal Cord Dysfunction.* This is seen in "low" paraplegics and spina bifida patients. The bladder has been disconnected from the spinal cord, and the patient is unable to feel fullness or initiate voiding. These patients can be rendered catheter free if there is no other mechanical impediment. They should be taught to manually empty their bladder (Crede maneuver) on a regular schedule.

5. *Incontinence of Mechanical Urethral Obstruction.* This group includes enlarged, prostrate, urethral stricture, etc.

The last three types of incontinence signal a possible life-threatening situation. This is because the distension and/or high pressures that can accompany these types of incontinence can create a *reverse flow* (reflux) of urine back toward the kidneys. Reverse urine flow produces pyelonephritis and hydronephrosis. These diseases can destroy kidney tissue and are the leading causes of death in spinal cord patients. Treatment is catheter drainage, which avoids high pressures or distension. Removal of the catheter, however desirable, should be undertaken only after careful study and with follow-up that includes periodic intravenous pyelograms.

Test for Types of Incontinence

Examine your comprehension of the previous material by answering the following:

1. *What is the goal of "bladder training?"*

_____

_____

2. *What normally happens to the urine, once in the bladder?*

_____

_____

_____

3. *Name four types of incontinence.*
   a. _____
   b. _____
   c. _____
   d. _____

4. *As presented in the material on overflow incontinence, describe reasons for caution in removing a catheter.*

_____

_____

_____

Answers: Your answers should correlate with these:

1. *The goal of bladder training is the emptying of the bladder as nearly normal as possible.*
2. *Once in the bladder, urine initiates the following chain of events.*
   a. *detrusor muscle fibers stretch,*
   b. *bladder wall tension increases to threshold level,*
   c. *sensory impulses go to the brain,*
   d. *motor impulses return to the bladder,*
   e. *detrusor muscle begins contraction waves, increasing bladder pressure,*
   f. *external sphincter reflexes,*

g. micturition reflex occurs,

h. bladder is allowed to empty.

3. a. Stress.

   b. Urge.

   c. Incontinence of high spinal cord dysfunction.

   d. Incontinence of low spinal cord dysfunction.

   e. Incontinence of mechanical urethral obstruction.

4. Patients diagnosed as having overflow incontinence are of clinical concern because of reflux (i.e., urine backing up the ureters), resulting in kidney infection and eventual destruction.

Information Gathering

We must begin to evaluate Mrs. Geriatric's existing condition of incontinence to begin formulating her care plan for bladder training.

From your education and experience, identify six pertinent questions you might ask when gathering information regarding the patient's voiding habits.

1. _____?
2. _____?
3. _____?
4. _____?
5. _____?
6. _____?

Compare your list of questions with the following:

1. How frequently does she void?
2. When is she incontinent?
3. What is her reaction to this incontinence?
4. Is she ever aware of the need to void? If so, how has she so indicated?
5. How much does she void?
6. Is there ever any dribbling involved?
7. Does she ever have urgency in voiding? If so, does she actually void then, or later?
8. Does she ever have difficulty initiating voiding?
9. Is her stream of force relatively normal?
10. What methods have proven effective in the past to assist her in voiding?
11. What is the character of her urine (e.g., are there signs of an existing infection from poor emptying)?
12. Does she or her family have any additional helpful information or suggestions?

If you listed any six of the above questions, we are in agreement. If you could not identify six appropriate questions, read this section again and think it over carefully before you proceed.

Bladder Training and Control

Bladder training can be initiated when:

1. the patient is alert enough to cooperate,
2. he is mobile enough to participate, and
3. he is catheter-free.

Frequently, the geriatric patient will have a catheter prior to the rehabilitation program to avoid overfilling of the bladder or incontinence. If possible, a catheter should eventually be removed as its presence *always* causes a bladder infection and can cause other complications such as pyelonephritis, bacteremia, and epididymitis. If the patient is unable to void effectively after catheter removal, it must be replaced after a reasonable time, to prevent discomfort, bladder overdistension, bacteremia, and reflux. If it is necessary to replace the catheter, an accurate measurement of bladder residual after voiding should be made to assist the physician in evaluating the problem.

Some physicians use intermittent clamping of the catheter. We do not recommend this technique because it does not increase the bladder's ability to contract, nor does it increase bladder capacity. It can also lead to complications.

Do not expect immediate control. It can take several days before real progress occurs, and *occasional* incontinence can persist much longer, or even permanently. If incontinence occurs at night, try having a scheduled time to offer a bedpan, urinal, or assistance to the bedside commode. Try to determine whether incontinence occurs at a specific time of the night and, if so, offer help just prior to it. Withholding or limiting fluids after the evening meal might help. When patients call for a bedpan it should be provided immediately if bladder training is to be effective. The physician could order a culture and sensitivity study and colony count of the urine to assist him in ordering antibiotic therapy if incontinence is secondary to infection.

Be aware of your patient's bladder capacity. If it was never more than 200 cc., it will not change simply because she is being bladder trained. If frequent assistance in voiding is required, be sure such help is available, offered, given, and understood by the nursing personnel.

Be sure to note the patient's awareness of the need to void. If it is diminished, she could need help and reminders, such as easy access to the commode, a nurse, or an alarm clock. Or, she might only need a watch or clock in easy view.

Initial attempts at voiding should be made hourly. Thereafter, time intervals should be gradually increased to four hours and progressed as the bladder tolerates. The usual nursing intervention techniques to initiate voiding should be used.

Remember that in order to void, urine must first be produced; therefore, fluids should be forced approximately one-half to one hour before attempting to void. Mrs. Geriatric could, at first, have residual that can go unnoticed if her voiding appears to be "quantity sufficient." Intake-output records facilitate accurate accounts of what the patient is doing.

Test for Bladder Training and Control

Answer the following questions:

1. *If noctural incontinence is prevalent, what might you do to help Mrs. Geriatric?*
    a. _____
    _____
    b. _____
    _____
    c. _____
    _____

2. *Identify two major factors that will affect her program.*
    a. _____
    b. _____

Answers:

1. a. *Withhold or limit fluids after dinner.*
    b. *Note usual time of occurrence, if any, and offer help before.*
    c. *Offer bedpan, urinal, or commode assistance at routine times.*
2. a. *Bladder capacity.*
    b. *Awareness of need to void.*

If your answers correspond to those given, please continue. If not, please review the appropriate section before you proceed.

Catheter Care

Correct catheter care is of utmost importance. It is very common for a urinary tract infection to occur secondary to ascending bacteria either through the catheter lumen or by way of the outer wall of the catheter. Therefore, it is imperative that perineal care be executed in a regular fashion. On the male it is recommended that three times a day the external urethral meatus should be cleansed with Betadine solution and then a thin film of Neosporin ointment applied around the external urethral meatus and on to the catheter as it exits from the urethra. On the female patient, the labia should be spread and washed with a mild soap and water detergent and then the area around the urethreal meatus should also be cleansed with Betadine solution. Neosporin ointment should then be applied at the meatus and on to the outside of the catheter as it exits from the external urethral meatus.

We do not recommend the use of continuous irrigation or routine irrigation of the Foley urethral catheter for several reasons. It is felt that a closed system is probably the safest system in inhibiting the development of urinary tract infections. The presence of a catheter causes a localized urinary tract infection; an open system for routine irrigation will introduce additional bacteria. Continuous irrigation with antibiotic irrigant is not routinely performed either. As soon as the irrigation is discontinued, the bladder is once again rapidly reinfected because of the presence of

Figure 8-2 **Sample Record of Urinary Bladder Training for One Week**

DATE	Sunday		Monday		Tuesday		Wednesday		Thursday		Friday		Saturday	
TIME	In-take	Out-put	In-take	Out-put	In-take	Out-put	In-take	Out-put	In-take	Out-put	In-take	Out-put	In-take	Out-put
6 a.m.	240cc													
7 a.m.		360cc												
8 a.m.	480cc													
9 a.m.		300cc												
10 a.m.	480cc													
11 a.m.		330cc												
12 noon	480cc	I												
1 p.m.		120cc												
2 p.m.	480cc													
3 p.m.		300cc												
4 p.m.	240cc													
5 p.m.		210cc												
6 p.m.	240cc													
7 p.m.		180cc												
8 p.m.														
9 p.m.-6 a.m.														

Total ounces   2640cc 1800cc
in 24 hours

Under "Intake" record (in c.c.) all fluids taken by mouth.
Under "Output" record (in c.c.) all urine passed. Record "I" for incontinence or accidental urinating.

Source: Form taken from *Nurses Can Give and Teach Rehabilitation* (New York: Springer Publishing, 1968).

the foreign body (Foley urethral catheter). If the catheter is not draining well or the patient is voiding around the catheter, the catheter should be irrigated under aseptic conditions with either a Toomey syringe or a bulb-type catheter syringe. The solution used to irrigate can be either normal saline or sterile water for irrigation.

If possible, the catheter used should ideally be one of the silastic type. This is inert and less apt to cause formation of infestation and bladder calculi as rapidly as the usual latex Foley catheter. In the male, the catheter should be taped to the abdomen to prevent pressure at the penile scrotal junction and prevent development of urethrocutaneous fistula.

The catheter should be changed every four to six weeks, depending on how it drains. When changing a catheter in the male, it is of utmost importance to be as atraumatic as possible to prevent injury to the prostatic urethra. The catheter should be well lubricated, and the penis should be held in a stretch position and on a slight angle, pointing toward the abdomen. The catheter balloon should never be blown up unless there is a return of urine from the lumen of the Foley catheter. If this is in question, one should irrigate the catheter prior to inflating the balloon.

Another important aspect is the urinary drainage bag. The bag should not be allowed to overfill, preventing drainage, which causes all the complications of an obstructed bladder.

Care Plan

You are now ready to formulate your own bladder training program care plan for Mrs. Geriatric. Study the sample in Figure 8-2 and use it as a guide in designing your plan.

When you have finished, take the Posttest.

- -

Posttest

1. *Answer the following as true or false by placing "T" or "F" in the blank by each statement.*

_____ a. *Bladder training is always effective.*

_____ b. *Bladder training refers to achievement of filling and emptying.*

_____ c. *Incontinence occurs when reflex emptying is uninhibited.*

_____ d. *Bladder training can begin any time and has little or no relation to the patient's medical condition.*

_____ e. *Cerebral control not only causes voluntary inhibition of voiding but voluntary initiation as well.*

_____ f. *Questioning the patient and family to determine a voiding history is not helpful in the bladder training program.*

_____ g. *Even though a bladder training program has been successful, occasional incontinence might occur.*

2. *Given a patient with a full bladder, place the following sequence of five steps in chronological order by numbering the statements in order of occurrence.*

Steps

_____ a. *Sensory impulses to the brain.*

_____ b. *Motor impulses return to the bladder.*

_____ c. *Detrusor muscle fibers stretch causing bladder wall tension.*

_____ d. *Detrusor muscle contracts.*

_____ e. *Bladder empties.*

3. *Circle the statements that apply to bladder training:*

a. *Patient's bladder capacity must be determined.*

b. *Nocturnal incontinence is almost inevitable and can rarely be corrected or diminished.*

c. *Scheduling times for voiding is useless; one must be ready for each voiding as it happens.*

d. *The patient's awareness of the need to void must be determined, and appropriate aids devised and used.*

e. *Hourly attempts at voiding are a good starting point, and progression from that is determined by bladder tolerance.*

f. *Withholding or limiting evening fluids can decrease incontinence at night.*

g. *Accurate intake-output records help to determine if large residual persists, which could cause infection from stagnation.*

Answers:

1. a. *False.*
   b. *True.*
   c. *True.*
   d. *False.*
   e. *True.*
   f. *False.*
   g. *True.*
2. *c*
   a
   b
   d
   e
3. *a, d, e, f.*

If you missed any of the posttest, you should review that section of this chapter.

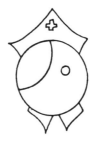

Pressure Sores: Development, Pathogenesis, Prevention, and Treatment

Robert D. Sine, M.D.

9.

Introduction and Objectives

Pressure sores can be a major problem for patients with various disabilities; therefore, the pathogenesis, prevention, and treatment of pressure sores are important components of the rehabilitation process. This chapter will assist you in accomplishing the following objectives:

1. understanding the pathogenesis of pressure sores,
2. recognizing conditions that might lead to the development of pressure sores,
3. recognizing some basic techniques and devices that can be used in the prevention of pressure sore development, and
4. identifying acceptable methods for treating pressure sores.

Pathogenesis of Decubiti

There should be no mystery surrounding pressure sores. The mechanism of their formation is well known. We are all vulnerable to sore formation and normally avoid them by moving, shifting (even in our sleep) in response to pain from weight-bearing areas starved of blood supply. This area is usually under a bony prominence where the pressure is highest. If we do not move off the area (as patients may not) the tissues caught between the bone and the surface eventually succumb (infarct) to the relative lack of metabolites. Necrosis takes place at all levels from skin to bone, although we might not be aware of it until the skin itself ulcerates and the dead tissue sloughs. This can take days.

The redness we see under points of pressure is a normal phenomenon known as hyperemia. The redness tells us that this is an area to be watched. However, it will disappear when the pressure is removed even when the tissue is doomed to necrosis. We cannot take comfort, therefore, when it returns to a normal appearance.

Check yourself to be sure we are off to a good start. Answer the following statements True or False. Then, correct any false answers in the space provided.

____ 1. *Despite medical advances, the mechanism of decubitus formation is shrouded in mystery.*
____ 2. *The contour of bony prominences protects against decubitus formation.*
____ 3. *The redness under a pressure point heralds impending ulceration.*
____ 4. *Friction is a major cause of ulcer formation.*

Answers:

All the above are false.

1. The mechanisms are well known.
2. Ulcer formation occurs under bony prominences.
3. The redness only signals a vulnerable area.
4. Friction does not play a role.

An ounce of decubitus prevention is worth many pounds of cure. Let's examine some preventive techniques.

Movement

The key concept in pressure sore prevention is to *restore movement!* We must live with pressures that are capable of sore production. The major defense, therefore, is relieving the pressure before the critical time has elapsed. This can only be done by the patient moving off the area. You should encourage as high a degree of mobility as is feasible in an effort to keep durations of pressure as short as possible. Unfortunately, due to their physical condition, many patients move only with difficulty. You must be alert in recognizing these patients. Most often, the immobile patient is one suffering from a neurological condition involving paralysis and/or loss of sensation (e.g., paraplegia, hemiplegia). However, the patient could be unconscious, heavily sedated, held down by apparatus, or so fearful of pain from a fracture site or arthritis that he chooses not to move.

You must help the patient weave continual movement back into his life. When planning and expediting patient care activities to prevent prolonged pressure on any one area, you should keep these points in mind:

1. An ambulatory patient should stay out of bed and move around as much as his condition permits.
2. Wheelchair-bound patients must be taught to relieve pressure from ischial tuberosities by doing wheelchair push-ups and by shifting weight in bed, even at night. It is better to lose a little sleep than to develop a pressure sore. You may even wish to teach patients to inspect hard-to-see pressure areas by using a mirror. The first three illustrations are examples of techniques for relieving pressure over ischial tuberosities.
3. To teach the patient to turn himself is your responsibility, but it is not enough. You must see that he does it. Therefore, you should plan individual positioning schedules for bed patients (such as the schedule in Figure 9-1). *Remember:* (a) the overall goal is self-care—the patient should learn to do this himself; (b) this is only a sample schedule and can be varied.

4. When a reddened area is noticed and the patient must be repositioned, the reddened area should be bridged. *Never* add more padding directly over the spot.
5. Setting the alarm clock at night is a good way to remind an alert patient to reposition himself. An alarm wrist watch is a good investment since it can be readily used during the day as well.
6. If a patient is to be discharged who you do not feel has learned to care for himself adequately and there is no Visiting Nurses Service available, you should ask the physician to defer discharge until self-care training is complete.

We know it must be the decision of individuals and treatment centers as to the methodology to be used in handling patient care activities, but we hope these suggestions are helpful.

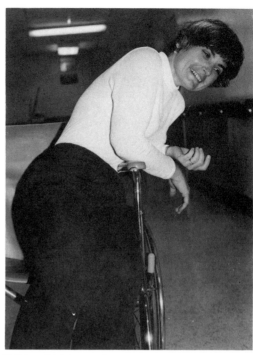

Shifting Weight—relieves pressure in patients who can't do wheelchair push-ups

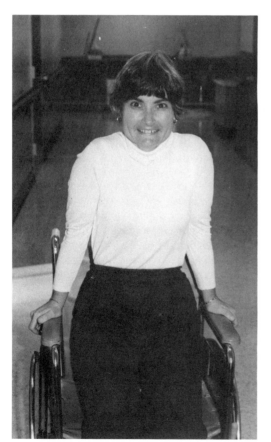

Wheelchair Push-Ups—maintain as long as possible.

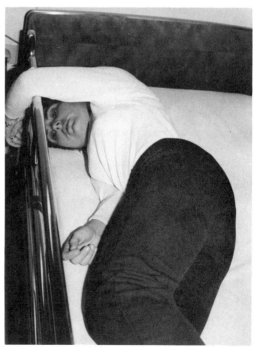

Using Side Rails

Figure 9-1   Sample Positioning Schedule for Patients on Complete Bed Rest

TURNING SCHEDULE

6:00 a.m.- 8:00 a.m.	left side—lying	breakfast—feeds self; bowel program every other day
8:00 a.m.-10:00 a.m.	supine	bed bath, including range of motion
10:00 a.m.-11:00 a.m.	prone	back care; work up tolerance, now tolerates 40 min. (turn to right)
11:00 a.m.- 1:00 p.m.	right side—lying	lunch—feeds self
1:00 p.m.-3:00 p.m.	left side—lying	visiting
3:00 p.m.- 4:00 p.m.	prone	back; range of motion; tolerates 40 min., try increase (turn to supine)
6:00 p.m.- 8:00 p.m.	right side—lying	dinner—feeds self visiting
8:00 p.m.-11:00 p.m.	left side—lying	evening care
11:00 p.m.- 3:00 a.m.	supine	sleeping
3:00 a.m.- 6:00 a.m.	right side—lying	sleeping

Positions that can be used:
  Supine
  Left and right side—lying
  Prone (build up tolerance)

Surface Modifications

Another less important technique for the prevention of pressure sores is to attempt to reduce pressure on vulnerable areas by modifying the surfaces in contact with these areas. They include efforts to distribute pressure more evenly and efforts to redistribute pressure. See the illustrations that follow.

Three important principles should be remembered when surface modifications are used:

1. They "buy time" in that they might delay the onset of tissue breakdown. Movement is still the key, however; and if the patient does not move, breakdown will still occur as there is still pressure. Do not be lulled into a false sense of security.

2. Sheets and dressings between the skin and the modification should be loose and soft or they could eliminate the effectiveness of the device, especially alternating air mattresses. It might look messy, but do not yield to the impulse to pull that sheet tight and smooth!

3. Do not add padding or other material under a bony prominence to raise it up. No matter how soft the material is, it will increase the pressure!

There are a large number of devices available commercially that, when applied intelligently and addressed to a patient's particular needs, can be helpful. None is a cure-all, and none will take the place of *fundamental nursing care,* which ensures movement.

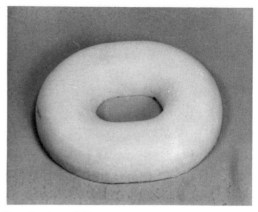

Doughnuts and Rings
Never use doughnuts for bridging, as they could increase edema.

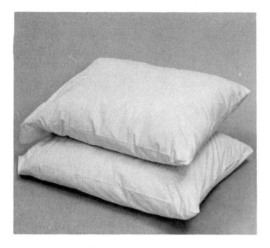

Pillows
Pillows—a must. (Note: The pillow under the head should be small and support only the head.)

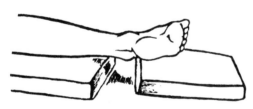

Foam Padding Bridging Ankle
Foam Padding has many uses: for bridging as shown here; also as seat cushions or back supports.

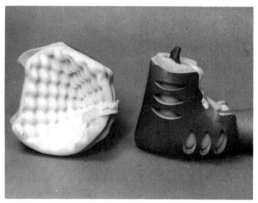

Spenko Stryker Boot
Spenko Stryker Boot is the best boot we know for preventing pressure on heels and lateral maleoli. It will also help keep foot aligned at a 90° angle.

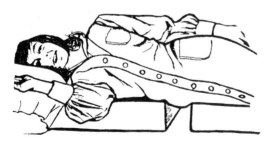

Foam Padding Bridging of Greater Tuberosity
Another way to use foam padding for bridging.

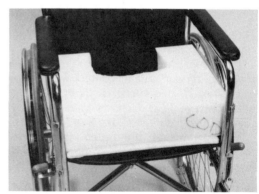

Horseshoe-Shaped Cushions
Most effective when used over seat board for reducing ischial tuberosity pressures.

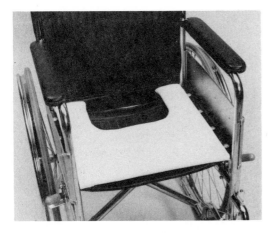

Seat Boards
Seat boards can be added to wheelchairs and are removable, making them more easily handled than a wheelchair with a solid seat.

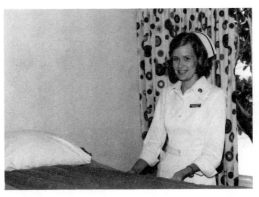

Water Beds
Inexpensive water beds can be made by filling an air mattress one-third full of water. Water beds are good to a point. Some patients get disoriented, and some get motion sickness; others tolerate them well. Avoid the use of pins and sharp objects—keep dry!

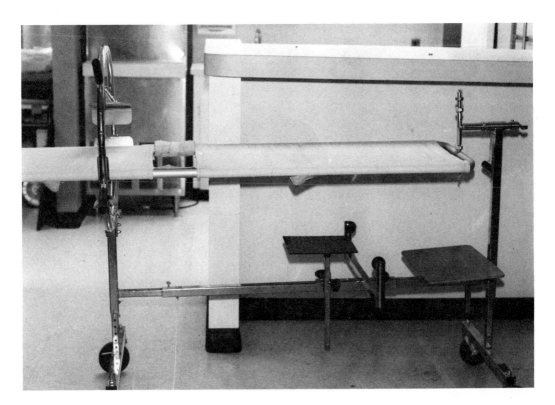

Turning Frames
Turning frames are very valuable in special cases (i.e., comatose patients). They should be discarded as early as possible, however, in favor of remobilization.

The following illustrations depict the areas under bony prominences vulnerable to breakdown. Study them so you can anticipate "trouble" spots.

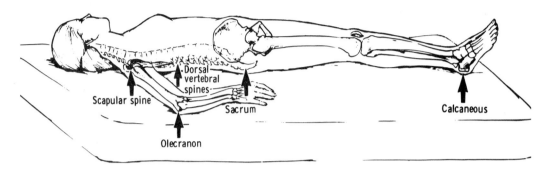

Supine Position

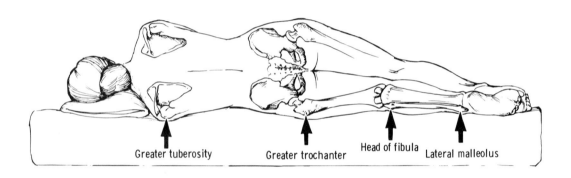

Sidelying

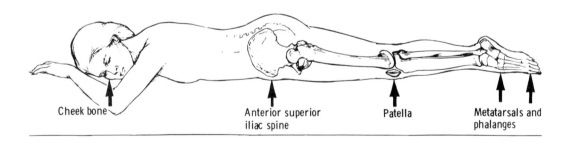

Prone Position

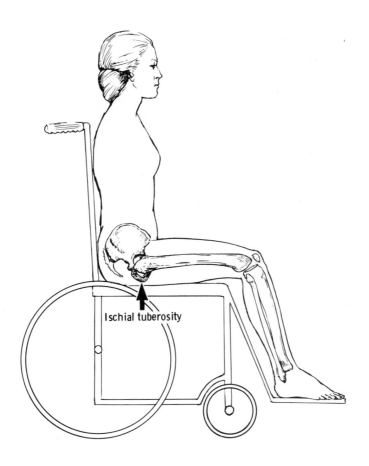

Sitting

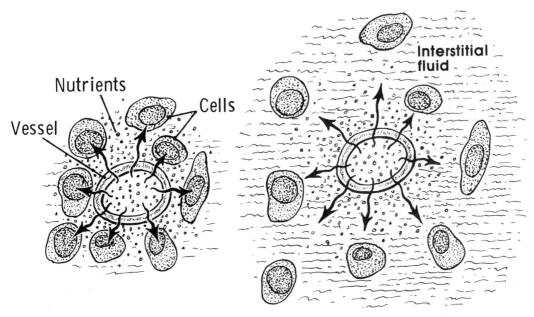

Normal

Edematous Tissue with Increased Interstitial Fluid

Treatable Conditions Predisposing to Decubiti

Any condition that reduces delivery of nutrients to the cell predisposes to decubiti development by reducing the time during which a given pressure can result in necrosis. These include:

1. Negative nitrogen balance. This can occur with sepsis, surgery, cancer, or simple inattention to nutrition. A high protein diet is often helpful, particularly in the early stages of paraplegia.
2. Anemia. This condition decreases oxygen delivery. It is easily diagnosed and usually responsive to treatment.
3. Edema. It is not usually appreciated how seriously edema interferes with the delivery of all nutrients. The presence of interstitial fluid increases the distance from capillary to cell. The rate of diffusion of nutrients is reduced by a square root of that distance. Even a minor amount of local edema can be a very important negative factor. (See illustrations on page 199.)

Healing

Decubiti are deep, wide wounds. Wound healing follows the same sequences irrespective of whether the wound was caused by pressure or some other trauma; yet "favorite" treatments for decubiti abound. Most are useless, and some certainly constitute harmful interference with the natural healing process.

Healing is a complex process involving migration of cells called fibroblasts into the area and a simultaneous chain of chemical reactions that change an exudate called *ground substance* into collagen. This complex combination of events eventually produces a highly vascular tissue known as *granulation tissue*, commonly seen at the bottoms of wounds. Such an involved and delicate process is vulnerable at many points to overzealous treatment, which could disrupt the sequence.

Another product of overtreatment is edema secondary to irritating agents. The negative effect of edema on nutrient delivery is as important in healing as it is in prevention.

As in all medical treatment, then—first the "don'ts" and then the do's."

1. Do not introduce any treatment or agent that could disrupt the healing sequence or irritate the tissues.
2. Do not allow pressures for durations that could reintroduce vascular insufficiency of tissue.
3. Do not interfere with the mobilization program. This might appear to conflict with number 2 above. It does not. Mobilization reduces the likelihood of *prolonged* pressure. There is no evidence that normal pressures, which include sitting pressures, for normal durations are of any danger. Additionally we have observed that decubiti often appear boggy and edematous and that patients who have been restricted to lying on their stomachs for over a year without results healed quickly when remobilized. It is likely that normal durations of normal pressure reduce edema, normalizing nutrient delivery and healing.
4. Observe daily. Watch for edema, purulence, undermining of skin, etc.
5. Cleanse gently but thoroughly with saline. Most necrotic tissue will slough with this alone. If pussy exudate persists, sugar sprinkled in the wound is probably the least irritating agent that will retard bacterial growth.
6. Persistance of adherent necrotic tissue might require surgical debridgement.
7. As in prevention, maintain nutrition, attend to anemia, and treat edema.

Occasionally the skin heals faster than the underlying tissue creating the danger of a sore being "roofed over." An apparently small decubitus will be found to be quite large when probed under the skin. An opening for drainage and reasonable cleansing can be maintained with loose packing using narrow iodoform gauze stripping. The underlying tissue will then fill in.

Another problem encountered is an underlying osteomyelitis. It is not uncommon, as necrosis usually dissects to the bone. It should be suspected whenever a decubitus refuses to heal. It can be diagnosed easily by x ray, and when treated the decubiti will begin to heal over it. Osteomyelitis must be thought of as there is often no other outward sign.

Surgery and/or grafting is most firmly indicated if the area seems in such poor condition that without a procedure future ulcerations are inevitable. Procedures might also be considered if they promise a shorter healing period without interfering with mobilization.

Decubiti theoretically should not, but will, occasionally appear even with the best of intentions and care. They should be the object of concern, but not despair, as they will heal if not interfered with by improper treatment or neglected. The tissues will fill in and reepithelialize in all but very large ulcers. A high protein diet will aid this process. We doubt that any of the numerous remedies that are topically applied affect the healing process, despite the claims of their proponents.

Remember that the job is not done until the patient can take care of himself. Only then can he be assured of freedom from sores after discharge.

Posttest

1. Pressure sustained for an abnormally long duration is the factor leading to pressure sore development. True or False
2. A decubitus ulcer—being of different origin than a wound of similar appearance—must be handled in a unique fashion. True or False
3. Pressure sores do not necessarily form in bed. True or False
4. Patients most prone to the development of pressure sores are those who do not perceive pain and those who cannot move when pain is perceived. True or False
5. The less the degree of pressure, the longer tissue can withstand it without infarction. True or False
6. The precautions applying to decubitus prevention also are applicable to healing. True or False
7. Any condition that slows or decreases the delivery of nutrients to the tissue predisposes toward formation and interferes with healing of decubiti. True or False
8. The prevention of pressure sores is an easy task. True or False

9. To cure a pressure sore is more difficult than to prevent one. True or False
10. Relief of pressure by movement soon enough to prevent the development of pressure sores is the best way we know to prevent them. True or False
11. It is dangerous to develop a sense of security through the use of surface modification. True or False
12. Pressure sore prevention must be the concern of all who work with chronically ill patients, and especially the alert patient himself. True or False
13. Decubiti are skin ulcers, and good skin care will prevent them. True or False
14. Antibiotics and debridgement are required for decubiti healing. True or False
15. The seriousness of decubiti requires that they take priority over other rehabilitation efforts, which should be stopped. True or False
16. Decubiti are not likely to heal without intensive treatment—the more intensive, the faster the healing. True or False

Answers

1. True.	9. True.
2. False.	10. True.
3. True.	11. True.
4. True.	12. True.
5. True.	13. False.
6. True.	14. False.
7. True.	15. False.
8. False.	16. False.

Results: The race is won, if you agree 100%, 80-100%, Very Good 0-79%, Suggest you review the chapter.

Suggested Readings

Colorado Public Health Service. *Elementary Rehabilitation Nursing Care*. Washington, D.C.: U.S. Government Printing Office, Public Health Service Publications No. 1436, April 1966.

Downey, John A., and Darling, Robert C. *Physiological Basis of Rehabilitation Medicine*. Philadelphia: W.B. Saunders Company, 1971.

Krusen, Frank H.; Kottke, Frederick J.; and Ellwood, Paul M. *Handbook of Physical Medicine and Rehabilitation.* 2nd ed. Philadelphia: W.B. Saunders Company, 1971.

Ma, Dong-Myung; Chu, D.S.; and Davis, S. "Pressure Relief Under The Ischial Tuberosities," *Archives of Physical Medicine and Rehabilitation* (July 1976).

Rossman, Isadore. *Clinical Geriatrics.* Philadelphia: J.B. Lippincott Company, 1972.

Stryker, Ruth. *Rehabilitation Aspects of Acute and Chronic Nursing Care.* Philadelphia: W.B. Saunders Company, 1972.

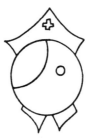

Utilizing Self-Instructional Materials in Rehabilitation Nursing Education

PAUL REPICKY, *Ph.D.*
PAMELA TRENT, *Ph.D.*
LEONARD HELLER, *Ed.D.*

10.

Introduction and Objectives

The format of the instructional program for this book involves the use of self-instructional materials that are enhanced through clinical instruction. The selection and modification of this teaching method were based on a consideration of *instructors'* capabilities and preferences, *students'* characteristics and availability, and the nature of the *subject matter*. Since you could have the opportunity to teach basic rehabilitation nursing techniques to other health professionals, the purpose of this chapter is to instruct you in the underlying rationale of this teaching method and the various techniques for its implementation.

The major emphasis of this self-instructional book is on the development of specific rehabilitation nursing skills, e.g., how to help hemiplegics dress themselves. The specific factual content was selected on the basis of its usefulness to learners in developing these basic skills. In placing an emphasis on skill development, one must be cautious of falling into the trap that surrounds the teaching of skills. That is, a program concentrating on skill development can easily be reduced to a *training* program, and such programs generally place little emphasis on the human component in learning. However, in the education of health professionals it is important to create an atmosphere in which the students feel that:

1. "Our instructors are really interested in us and our learning," and similarly
2. "Our patients' feelings and thoughts are very important for us to consider."

It is essential to develop these attitudes because they will affect health professionals' willingness to learn as well as their interactions with patients.[1] A positive rapport between patients and health care professionals is especially significant in the area of rehabilitation, where cooperation and effort are the cornerstones to growth.

At the completion of this chapter you should be able to:

1. Identify and justify the key elements of the self-instructional materials used in this book.
2. Design effective clinical experiences for the sections in this book.
3. Evaluate your instruction by assessing its effects on student performance, student attitude, and the quality of rehabilitation care being delivered to patients.

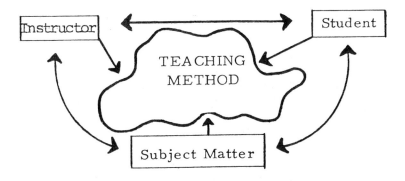

Self-Instructional Materials

Self-instructional materials are designed to provide a self-directed pattern of study for the learner. They can be used as part of an ongoing program or in isolation. In any case, the materials must be prepared so the various roles of the teacher (i.e., questioning, identifying problems, rewarding, etc.) are fulfilled.

As you might have noticed, the self-instructional sections in this book have several common elements: objectives, feedback loops, self-pacing, posttests, and a different style of presentation.

Objectives: "Where are we going?"

The major consideration in defining objectives is to specify, as precisely as possible, what the student should be able to *do* as a result of the instruction. Examine the following objectives. Which one more clearly identifies what the student should be able to do?

1. To appreciate the utility of self-care techniques for hemiplegic patients.
2. To select appropriate self-help devices for use by hemiplegic patients.

What does it mean to "appreciate the utility of?" This phrase can be interpreted in many ways. But, "select appropriate self-help devices" is a more precise description because it defines a clearly observable behavior.

Many objectives of health professions education programs are relatively easy to specify because most of the techniques, skills, and knowledge required of the learner can be identified by the instructor. For example, psychomotor skills (e.g., pulse taking) are frequently part of a health professions curriculum and can be clearly defined.

Once the objectives have been formulated, it is important to keep them clearly in mind throughout the instructional program. They can be useful as a means of organizing material for presentation, establishing expectations of students, and informing students of what lies ahead. In addition, evaluation can follow directly from a set of clearly defined objectives (refer to the "Evaluation" section).

Feedback Loops: "I'd Really Be Lost If I Didn't Know I Was Lost!"

Since, in self-instruction, the teacher is not available to recognize any problems in the student's progress, the instructional materials must perform this function. This is done through the use of a series of internal checks or "feedback loops," which are built into the chapters. These feedback loops are in the form of small quizzes that assess the learner's comprehension and retention of material.

The questions in the feedback loops are designed to emphasize the important points of the instruction and to help the students identify the areas in which they are developing inaccurate concepts or knowledge. Students must recognize this function so they will not be disheartened by their errors. They should use this information to make their learning more effective.

Self Paced: "Now I've Got It!"

One great advantage of self-instructional materials is that the students can use them at a place, time, and pace that are most comfortable. This is possible since the materials are portable, and a teacher need not regulate the pace of the learning. This allows students of all capabilities to complete the instruction successfully.

Posttest: "How Do I Know When I Have Arrived?"

The brief test following each chapter is designed to let the students know what they have and have not mastered. Students should analyze their incorrect responses to determine which concepts or knowledge areas they need to review. Thus, the test becomes a learning device rather than a threatening, evaluation instrument.

Self-instructional materials are designed differently from the usual textbook presentations. This is a function of: (1) a writing style that utilizes humor and a conversational tone; (2) feedback loops that signify the successful completion of a section; and (3) involving the students in hypothetical problem-solving. This moves them beyond passive reading of textbook expositions and closer to the real experience.

Test for Self-Instructional Materials

Now let's see what you have learned. Please answer the following questions.

1. *What is the purpose of this set of questions?* _____

   _____

2. *Thus far, in this chapter you have completed which objective? No.* _____

3. *Do you think that the self-paced design of this instructional program has been helpful to you as a learner?*_____

   Why or why not? _____

   _____

   _____

4. *If a student incorrectly answered several questions presented as part of a feedback loop, what alternative procedure might he/she follow to improve his/her comprehension of that section (other than reviewing the same material)?*_____

   _____

   _____

   _____

Answers:

1. *Give you an indication of how well you comprehended the previous section. (It is part of a feedback loop.)*

2. *One.*

3. *(There's no one "right" answer to this question. You had to think a little to answer it. This is the kind of question that, when it is appropriate, should be asked of your students.)*

4. *(You have been challenged again!) You might have answered:*

   a. *she might research the topic further using various resources, or*

   b. *she might seek help from an instructor or another individual who is knowledgeable in that area, or*

   c. *if the chapter were designed differently, it might have provided additional instruction in each section approaching the topic from a different point of view, or, etc.*

When you are satisfied with your performance in this section, please continue.

Designing Clinical Instruction as a Supplement to Self-Instructional Materials

The purpose of designing clinical instruction is to provide your students with practical experiences that augment the material presented in the self-instructional chapters. This experience enables students to apply specific skills and knowledge in "simulated" situations. In general, the application of skills and knowledge enhances the students' ability to conceptualize the written materials; that is, they "learn by doing."

In conjunction with this self-instructional program you might wish to design clinical experiences for your students. If you are employed in a clinical setting, designing experiences of this type should be relatively easy. The following specific guidelines are offered to assist you:

1. You may use the objectives designed for the self-instructional program or modify them slightly for the clinical setting. Basically, any objective you use should be a clear, concise statement of what the students should be able to do as a result of your instruction. Make every effort to ensure that your students understand the objectives at the start of the instruction and to remind them of those objectives throughout the clinical experience.
2. You should define the smaller tasks that make up the larger, overall skill you wish to teach. Then, design the clinical situation in terms of a step-by-step progression of smaller tasks. Be certain that your students are able to perform each preliminary task adequately before proceeding to more complex tasks. (Remember the Progressive Mobilization Staircase, where the patient built his strength and mobility through successive steps?)
3. You might wish to try a simulated experience with your students before allow-

ing them to use a skill in a real situation. The purpose of a simulation is to involve the students in an experience that closely approximates a real-life situation. For instance, you might give them an opportunity to practice tasks and skills on plastic models, friends, other health personnel, etc. The advantages of using a simulated experience are as follows:
a. a controlled situation can be arranged;
b. the situation can be reenacted repeatedly;
c. it presents a "hands on" experience to the student (i.e., the student can manipulate materials); and,
d. mistakes can be made without injuring a patient.

The major disadvantage, of course, is that a simulated experience is still not "real." However, the purpose of this teaching technique is to provide an experience that will allow the students to progress safely and confidently from written instruction to the actual implementation of skills.

4. It is important that the clinical experience be organized in a manner that reinforces the self-instructional materials. For instance, recall the instructional chapter that described the steps involved in teaching a hemiplegic patient to dress himself. When you are presenting that set of skills in a clinical experience, you might allow the students to practice the dressing procedures themselves.
5. If equipment is needed you should thoroughly familiarize the students with it. You might want them to handle and even try using it. You might feel that this is an obvious guideline; however, it is frequently overlooked.

The Human Element

Remember, your students are human. They might demand not only your time and expertise but also a great deal of patience and understanding, especially in the clinical situation. They are learning new skills to help other people; acquiring these skills will not be uniformly easy for all of them. To facilitate their learning you might:

1. Reward and encourage their efforts to learn. Provide sincere verbal praise and/or nonverbal recognition for each student's efforts. Showing that you care about their learning will go a long way in stimulating their desire to learn.
2. Accept and use their wrong answers. When students make errors you should reward them for their effort and help them to analyze the reason(s) for their mistakes. Thus, rather than admonish them you can create a positive learning experience from an incorrect response.
3. Deemphasize the negative. Avoid the use of sarcasm or demeaning your students' attempts to learn.

Questioning Techniques

Your effectiveness as an instructor, particularly in the clinical setting, will be greatly enhanced if you continually work on the development of your questioning techniques. Interpretations of educational research have shown that, generally, the kind of answer a student gives is directly related to the kind of question that is asked. Sounds obvious, right?

What kinds of questions will you ask in your clinical instruction? As an instructor, you should be aware of the complexity of your questions. A good way to determine the level of complexity is to ask yourself, "What kinds of intellectual operations must a student perform to answer my question?"

It might help you to classify your questions into one of the following broad categories:

1. *Knowledge questions* can be answered by simple recall of information. For example, "What is hemianopsia?", and "What are the characteristics exhibited by hemiplegic patients?"
2. *Convergent questions* have one correct answer and require the student to do more than recall information. For example, "Your patient has the following problems: *x, y,* and *z.* Which wheelchair adaptations will he need?"
3. *Divergent questions* have more than one correct answer. For example, "If your patient is depressed, what might you do to cheer him up?"
4. *Evaluative questions* require the student to evaluate a situation and give his/her

opinion—many answers are possible. For example, "Do you think it is important for your patient to do active ROM exercises? Why or why not?"

Please do not feel that you need to classify every question before you ask it. Just keep in mind the fact that questions at different levels require the student to perform different mental operations. It is advised that you *ask questions at all levels of complexity* and, in particular, get your students to think and respond beyond the simple recall level. To accomplish this it might help to ask questions in a sequential order. That is, ask low level (knowledge or convergent) questions about a topic before proceeding to higher level (divergent or evaluative) questions. Furthermore, you must realize that formulating an answer to a high level question takes more time. So, be patient; give your students *time to think!*

Now it is time to try an exercise that challenges you to design a clinical experience for your students. First, choose a specific skill from among the various rehabilitation techniques presented in the previous chapters. Then, design an appropriate experience in terms of the guidelines presented above. This is only a small, practical exercise—so be as brief as possible. An outline has been provided to guide you. (Remember to incorporate thought-provoking questions where appropriate.)

1. *List the objectives. Remember to make them as specific as possible so you can determine when they have been accomplished successfully.*

_____
_____
_____
_____

2. *Explain the skill. List the specific tasks that must be achieved.*

_____
_____
_____

3. *Design a simulation that will help the students learn the skill. Explain the purpose of the simulation.*

_____
_____
_____
_____

4. *Give a brief description of how you will organize the clinical experience.*
   Step 1 _____
   Step 2 _____
   _____
   etc.
5. *Describe the equipment and tell how it will be used in the clinical experience.* _____
   _____
   _____
   _____

Please evaluate your responses to this practice exercise on the basis of the guidelines presented in this section.

Evaluation

Now you will want to determine whether your program has been effective. This will help you to decide whether the self-instruction and/or the clinical instruction need to be improved and whether the objectives have been met. This is where clearly stated objectives can aid greatly in the evaluation process. That is, the description of what students should be able to do provides an appropriate, ready-made criterion for evaluation. If the students can do what is described in the objectives, the instruction was effective.

In evaluating the level of effectiveness, you should assess three factors:

1. the students' comprehension of the information contained in the self-instructional packages;
2. the students' ability to perform the skills in a real situation; and
3. the degree to which your students' delivery of health care has been improved.

Evaluation of these three factors will vary in difficulty. For instance, it is qualitatively easier to determine whether the students remember specific information than it is to determine if health care has been improved. Two evaluation strategies that you can use in *your* setting are a *pretest/posttest design* and a *participant observation* technique.

Pretest/Posttest Design

The pretest/posttest evaluation design can be used to assess the students' comprehension of information. According to this design,

similar tests are administered before and after the entire self-instructional program. Both the pretest and posttest contain questions about conceptual and factual information presented in the program. The students' scores on these tests indicate their comprehension of that information. For example, if a 100-item multiple choice test is given at the beginning of a program and administered again at the end, the two scores (pretest and posttest) will measure comprehension of the information contained in the program prior to and following completion of the program. The positive difference between these scores is a measure of what was learned.

Participant Observation

The participant observation technique* can be used to determine the level of adequacy in performing a skill and the degree to which health care has been improved. This technique depends on the evaluator's sensitivity and insight. When you evaluate in this manner you become a researcher who both participates and observes in the setting. As a participant you will be personally and subjectively involved with the individuals in the setting; as an observer you will remain objective enough to analyze the cues, which tell you about the adequacy with which a skill is performed and the types of improvements that have been made in the health care setting.

In the case of observation, Emily Mumford and James K. Skipper state,[2] "One special factor that frequently seems to characterize the superb nurse, the brilliant physician, the writer of genius, the creative scientist, is a special ability to observe accurately and clearly in his (her) special field of interest." No doubt, you are aware of the importance of this ability, but did you know that this ability is a skill that can be developed?

One way of developing the observation skill is by learning to focus your attention on meaningful detail and then to record what you

---

*Participant observation is a technique that has been utilized by anthropologists for studying various cultures and by sociologists for studying social milieux. It is recently being utilized in studies of organizational settings. Although the technique is simplistically defined here, it has broader implications and requirements for more involved research studies.

observed. You will find that you become increasingly more adept at picking out important, subtle cues. Once these cues are recorded in a systematic fashion, and then analyzed, you will be able to see a larger picture of the situation. For instance, if you want to know whether your students can perform a specific skill, you could unobtrusively observe their ability to accomplish specific tasks while in the health care setting, instead of putting them through a prescribed testing situation. If you record your perceptions of the student's performance, it will provide you with information for a total view of the situation as well as with documentary evidence about the level of achievement.

To develop *your* observational skills, it is recommended that you keep a diary (journal, field notes, log, etc.) of your observations. Write down pertinent information about your students' ability to perform certain skills in the real situation and about the types of improvements that have been made in the health care setting. This information should include the following observation categories:

1. *Place:* location of the action in the health care setting (e.g., office, hall, ward, etc.).
2. *Time* the action takes place: time of day (clock time), duration of action (clock time), and date of observation.
3. *Participants* in the action: names and/or titles of participants in the action.
4. *Event* or content of the interaction: verbal behavior, verbatim content, loaded words; nonverbal behavior, facial expressions, body movements. Both should include (1) what happened and (2) behaviors that indicate participants' reactions to what happened.
5. *Observer:* reactions to what happened at the time, and reactions to what happened in retrospect. Included here are (1) observer's feelings, (2) interpretations made

at the time, and (3) subsequent interpretations.

To cover these categories comprehensively, you might organize your notes according to the design in Figure 10-1. (This is only a suggestion since everyone has a unique way of organizing information.) Now, let's consider an example of how you might record your observations. We will begin with a scenario.

Scenario: Through self-instructional materials and clinical instruction you have taught Basic Rehabilitation Nursing Techniques to Nurse P.J. It just so happens that P.J. is stationed in your ward, and you are able to observe her interactions with various patients. You are also involved with P.J. and the patients on a personal level because you interact with them daily. Thus, you receive verbal comments about a wide range of everyday activities.

For the most part, the ward has a congenial atmosphere and it is like one big happy family. The only exception is a very depressed, middle-aged male who had a mild stroke that left him forgetful and weak. He seems to be growing weaker and more withdrawn as the days go by. In the past, the health personnel approached him with cheerful smiles but helped the man only with necessary functions, i.e., changing bedding, cleaning. But now you notice that Nurse P.J. has been interacting with the man on a different basis.

Examine your hypothetical observations in the diary shown in Figure 10-1.

Figure 10-1   Diary of Your Observations

PLACE AND TIME	PARTICIPANTS	EVENT (CONTENT OF INTERACTION)	OBSERVER REACTIONS
Ward A - between Mr. Z.'s room and the hall 9:32 a.m.	Nurse P.J.	(I am watching outside the room) Nurse P.J. enters room. Her eyes are bright and she is smiling. She says to Mr. Z., "What a nice day for you to learn to wash behind your shoulder. I will get things ready." Mr. Z. groans a little.	Hummm. This is interesting. The nurses usually wash him.
Mr. Z.'s room 9:40 a.m.	Nurse P.J. Mr. Z.	P.J. says, in an encouraging tone, "Remember how you learned to dangle your legs on the side of the bed yesterday? And how you learned to sit up for awhile?" Mr. Z. nods with a semi-smile on his face. P. J. says, "Good, today you are going to reach your arm up and wash behind your shoulder."	She is really getting into this rehabilitation stuff. I like this.
Hallway - 9:45 a.m.	Me	I leave room to return to hall desk.	
Hallway - 10:30 a.m.	Mr. and Mrs. Z.	Mr. Z. is in wheelchair. Although *he* still has a little bit of sadness in his look, Mrs. Z. is smiling.	Well, he's finally out of bed! How wonderful!
Mr. Z.'s room 12:30 p.m.	Mr. and Mrs. Z.	(I just walked past Mr. Z.'s room to peek in.) This is lunch time and Mrs. Z. is feeding Mr. Z. as usual.	Mr. Z. seems very apathetic. He's just accepting the food and not indicating any emotions.
Mr. Z.'s room 12:35 p.m.	Mr. and Mrs. Z. P.J.	(I'm in corridor and I hear P.J. Her tone is happy and hopeful.) "Hey, Mr. Z.! Every day you have been learning a little more. You've been slowly building your strength so you can completely care for yourself again. Why don't we take another step today, let you feed yourself. Come on Mrs. Z., you can help."	She includes Mrs. Z.... good. Wow! I am certainly happy that P.J. took that rehabilitation course. Perhaps we can get more instructional packages and teach these rehabilitation concepts and skills to everyone. Now P.J. can help us teach others.

(continued on next page)

PLACE AND TIME	PARTICIPANTS	EVENT (CONTENT OF INTERACTION)	OBSERVER REATIONS
Mr. Z.'s room 12:45 p.m.	Mr. and Mrs. Z. P.J.	I peeked in again and saw Mr. Z. holding a spoon. He had a smile on his face and a twinkle in his eye. Mrs. Z. is smiling, too. P.J. is getting ready to leave the room. She approaches the door. Oops. . . she saw me watching.	I am so very pleased about Mr. Z.'s progress that it is hard to keep notes.

and so on . . . get the idea?

Now is the time to test yourself on your comprehension of the material in this section. In the space at the left, indicate whether each statement is True (T) or False (F).

____1. In determining whether instruction has been effective in the Basic Rehabilitation Nursing Techniques course, you need to consider only one factor—that is, the amount of information that has been retained from the instructional chapters.

____2. Determining the level of instructional effectiveness will help you know whether the instruction needs to be altered or improved and whether the objectives have been met.

____3. Using a pretest/posttest design in evaluating the course will provide evidence about the degree to which health care has been improved in a particular setting.

____4. Observation is an art and cannot be developed as a skill.

____5. Participant observation is a technique for assessment that depends on the student's sensitivities and insights.

____6. In the participant observation technique, observation and recording go hand in hand.

____7. These five observation categories were identified for use in the participant observation technique: (a) place, (b) time, (c) participants, (d) event, (e) observer.

Answers:

1. False.
2. True.
3. False.
4. False.
5. False.
6. True.
7. True.

If you answered two or more incorrectly, please review the chapter. Otherwise continue to the posttest for this chapter.

Posttest

Please complete or answer all of the following statements and questions. Check your answers with those provided at the end of the posttest.

1. To design an effective instructional program one must carefully consider these three important variables: _____ , _____ , and _____ .
2. Why might objectives be particularly useful in the education of health professionals? _____
   _____
   _____

3. The posttest at the end of each self-instructional package should be used to help identify those areas that the learner does and does not understand. True or False

4. One good way to get your students to think at higher intellectual levels is to _____
_____

5. Five guidelines that should be followed in setting up a clinical experience for students are:

    a. _____

    b. _____

    c. _____

    d. _____

    e. _____

6. You can expect that learning the basic skills will be uniformly easy for all your students. *True or False*

7. Giving reward and encouragement is not really important when dealing with students but is extremely important when you interact with patients. *True or False*

8. Evaluating the effectiveness of the instruction will help you to know what?

    a. _____

    b. _____

9. Two evaluation strategies that can be used in your educational setting are:

    a. _____

    b. _____

10. Observation is a skill that can be developed. *True or False*

Answers. Compare your answers with these.

1. The student, the instructor, the subject matter.
2. Several correct answers are possible. Two possibilities are:
    ____Many of the skills and concepts to be learned can be identified by the instructor.
    ____The objectives (particularly psychomotor objectives) can be clearly specified.
3. True.
4. Ask them higher level questions.
5. a. List objectives clearly and concisely.
    b. Explain the skill and list the tasks.
    c. Design a simulation.
    d. Organize the clinical experience in such a way as to reinforce the instructional materials.
    e. Familiarize the student with necessary equipment.
6. False.
7. False.
8. a. If the instruction needs to be improved.
    b. If the objectives have been met.
9. a. Pretest/posttest design.
    b. Participant observation technique.
10. True.

If you answered seven or more questions correctly you have done well. If not, review the appropriate section(s) of this chapter or consult with your instructor.

When you are satisfied that you understand the material in this chapter...

CONGRATULATIONS !
YOU HAVE COMPLETED THIS
BOOK!

Good luck, and do not forget to use your newly acquired nursing and teaching skills.

Notes

Carl Rogers, *Freedom to Learn* (Columbus, Ohio: Charles Merrill, 1969).
Emily Mumford and James K. Skipper, *Sociology In the Hospital* (New York: Harper and Row, 1967), p. 71.

Epilogue

In attempting to write a statement on my philosophy of Rehabilitation Nursing, I present three patients. Each of you knows at least one of them.

- A twenty-one-year-old married woman was involved in an automobile accident and sustained serious head and neck injuries. After the acute phase of her illness, she was left with right hemiplegia, aphasia, and a tracheotomy.
- A fourteen-year-old boy received a spinal cord injury from a motorcycle accident. He survived but had muscle spasticity, which forced his body into a fetal position.
- An eighty-three-year-old greatgrandmother, alert and active, fell at home and fractured her left hip. She tolerated surgical repair well, but postoperatively she was confused and very weak.

These patients and many like them who have suffered disabling illness or injury benefited from the advanced techniques medical science provided them. Time, indeed years, has probably been added to their lives. But what of the quality of those years? Will they be spent as "helpless invalids" or "bedridden patients" dependent on other people even for the simplest life-sustaining activities? Or will these people be able to live at the highest level of function within the limitations of their disabilities? It is hoped that the latter will be the ultimate picture. But what can be done to accomplish this? The answer is Physical Rehabilitation, a discipline that seeks to add breadth and meaning as well as length to the patient's life. When an individual learns self-sufficiency, that person acquires dignity.

In restoring usefulness, a sense of purpose can be found. If people seek to broaden their horizons, they generally find new interests. Such people cannot be described as "invalid," regardless of the disability.

Simply, the idea behind all rehabilitation techniques is to teach and encourage the patient to do as much as possibly can be done by the patient alone, offering minimal assistance and firm reassurance. This demands patience as well as skill. How much easier it is for you to button a patient's shirt rather than just stand by for ten long minutes, watching him struggle to button it while you can only offer encouragement. Bedrest itself can be the cause of severe disability or death. Thus, Progressive Mobilization—getting the patient *out of bed*— is initially the essential ingredient to successful rehabilitation.

Unfortunately, these ideas and concepts are often diametrically opposed to the old-fashioned, traditional images of nursing care. They are also not being taught well enough to undergraduate nursing students and other hospital personnel, and implementing these ideas requires enormous patience and an array of new skills. All of this is, however, amply rewarded by the experience of discharging a patient you've helped to regain independence and self-esteem.

Restoration of purpose and function is a noble cause. But is it realistic? Can it be done? Yes! The techniques and suggestions offered in this text told you *how*! They work. Patients get better faster. That's my philosophy of rehabilitation nursing. And that is what this book is all about—translating philosophy into action. It is hoped that the three patients described above will be cared for by people who espouse this philosophy and who practice the techniques presented in this book.

Marie B. Campbell, R.N.

Contributors' Profiles

Ruth Avidan, O.T.R., is a Registered Occupational Therapist trained at the Israel School of Physical Therapy in Jerusalem, Israel. Mrs. Avidan was, during the course of the initial stages of the development of this book, Chief of Occupational Therapy at Rosewood General Hospital's Rehabilitation Unit in Houston, Texas. At the time of the writing of this book, Mrs. Avidan resided in Israel.

Marie Benoit Campbell, R.N., is Head Nurse of the Physical Rehabilitation Unit of Rosewood General Hospital, Houston, Texas. She came to Rosewood as a graduate of the Memorial Hospital School of Nursing in Worcester, Massachusetts. Mrs. Campbell has ten years experience in the field of Acute Care Nursing. For the last four years, Mrs. Campbell has been directly involved in Intensive Rehabilitation Nursing.

Joanna B. Chase, M.A., was Supervisor of Speech Pathology Services, Rosewood General Hospital, Houston, Texas, where she was responsible for the evaluation and treatment of patients with communication disorders. She holds the Certificate of Clinical Competence from the American Speech and Hearing Association and is listed on the registry of the International Association of Laryngectomees as a certified instructor of alaryngeal speech.

Leonard E. Heller, Ed.D., is Director, Office of Medical Education, College of Medicine,

University of Kentucky. He has served as Assistant Director of the Office of Educational Resources and Research at the University of Michigan, College of Medicine, and as Coordinator of Evaluation, Center for Allied Health Manpower Development, Baylor College of Medicine. Dr. Heller is an educational consultant for curriculum design and program evaluation to various allied health programs.

J. David Holcomb, Ed.D., is Associate Director of the Center for Allied Health Manpower Development, Baylor College of Medicine, and Director of Allied Health Education, Veterans Administration Hospital, Houston, Texas. He is an Assistant Professor of Allied Health Sciences at Baylor and is a member of the faculties of Texas A&M University, the University of Houston, and the University of Texas. He serves as the Project Director of Baylor's Allied Health Teacher Education and Administrative Leadership Program. Dr. Holcomb is the coauthor of a book on improving medical education.

Jane Jester, M.S.W., is a social worker with Sheltering Arms of Houston, Texas, a counseling agency for people 60 years old and over. She has served as a medical social worker for Rosewood General Hospital, where she worked primarily with rehabilitation patients. She has been a part-time instructor in the Department of Sociology, Houston Baptist University.

Virginia L. Kerr, O.T.R., was, until recently, the head of Occupational Therapy in the Rehabilitation Unit, Rosewood General Hospital, Houston, Texas. A 1970 graduate of Texas Woman's University, Mrs. Kerr was an occupational therapist at Rosewood for the past six years.

Shelly E. Liss, M.D., is Director of the Department of Physical Medicine and Rehabilitation, Memorial Hospital, Houston, Texas, and Clinical Assistant Professor, Department of Physical Medicine, Baylor College of Medicine. He is an active spokesman for the field of Rehabilitation Medicine in numerous local, state, and national organizations and has been responsible for the development of several statewide programs utilizing rehabilitation techniques for general and patient populations. Dr. Liss' publications include papers demonstrating how the medical profession can use rehabilitation techniques to improve patient care in various diagnostic categories.

Paul A. Repicky, Ph.D., is a Research Associate in the Division of Research in Medical Education, University of Southern California School of Medicine, Los Angeles. Currently, he is Coordinator of the Physician Extender Reimbursement Study surveying Nurse Practitioners, Physician's Assistants, and Medex in the U.S. In 1974-75, he was a postdoctoral fellow at the Center for Allied Health Manpower Development, Baylor College of Medicine. During his fellowship year, Dr. Repicky coordinated the Basic Rehabilitation Techniques Project for Baylor College of Medicine and Rosewood General Hospital.

Robert E. Roush, Ed.D., is Director, Center for Allied Health Manpower Development, and Head, Division of Allied Health Sciences,

Department of Community Medicine, Baylor College of Medicine. He coordinates training programs from the high school to postgraduate level and directs educational research on the preventive aspects of cardiovascular disease. Dr. Roush has completed postdoctoral work in medical education and public health, respectively, at the University of Southern California School of Medicine and The University of Texas School of Public Health. Additionally, he is also a member of the Adjunct Graduate Faculties of The University of Houston and Texas A&M University.

Robert D. Sine, M.D., is Chief, Department of Rehabilitation Medicine at St. Mary's Hospital, San Francisco, California. He was formerly Director of the Rehabilitation Medicine Department, Rosewood General Hospital, Houston, Texas, and Clinical Assistant Professor, Department of Physical Medicine, Baylor Còllege of Medicine. He is active in the leadership of his state specialty society and an expert in the fields of rehabilitation and electrodiagnosis.

Ruth Stryker-Gordon, R.N., M.A., is Assistant Professor and Assistant Coordinator of the Center for Long Term Care Administration Education at the University of Minnesota. She was Director of Nursing Education at Sister Kenny Rehabilitation Institute for six years. She is the author of many articles and several books, one of which is on rehabilitative nursing and is cited as a resource in several chapters of this book.

Pamela J. Trent, Ph.D., is Assistant Professor of Medical Education, University of Illinois Medical Center, Chicago, Illinois. Her responsibilities include teaching, consulting, and research in the areas of organizational and faculty development, health professions education and evaluation, and research design. She was formerly a postdoctoral fellow at the Center for Allied Health Manpower Development, Baylor College of Medicine. During her fellowship year, Dr. Trent assisted in the coordination of the Basic Rehabilitation Techniques Project for Baylor College of Medicine and Rosewood General Hospital.

Georgianna Burbidge Wilson, L.P.T., is currently Chief of Physical Therapy in the Rehabilitation Unit, Rosewood General Hospital, Houston, Texas. She is a 1966 graduate of the Mayo Clinic School of Physical Therapy. Mrs. Wilson has previously worked in California at the Contra Costa County Hospital Rehabilitation Center with Dr. Gerald Hirschberg, originator of the Stand-up, Step-up Program, and has been influential in its development at Rosewood. She also assisted in the coordination of and taught in the Basic Rehabilitation Techniques workshops presented at Rosewood.

Index

A

Abscess, 3
Activities of daily living (ADL), 4, 129, 130, 143, 148, 155, 156
  book holder, 143
  card holder, 144
  card playing, 144
  card shuffler, automatic, 144
  cut-out window, 144
  homemaking and work simplifications, 145
  reading, 143-144
  sewing, 144
  telephone, 144
  writing, 144
  See also Parkinsonism
Alphabet card, 111
  See also Dysarthria
Ambulation, 6, 8, 9
American Cancer Society—Reach to Recovery, 123
American Heart Association, 123, 145, 153
  See also Activities of daily living (ADL); Homemaking and Work Simplifications
American Speech and Hearing Association, 110
Ankles, area to be positioned, *35*
  foot boards, 36
Antimalarials, 12
Aphasia, 3, 7, 112, 215
  dysarthria, 112
  emotional lability, 112
  fatigue, 112
  hemianopsia, 112
  language symbols, 112
  memory impairment, 112
  reduced attention span, 112
Arms and hands, area to be positioned, 36
Arterio-venous malformation, 3
Arthritis, 2, 11, 12, 14, 32, 128
  management of, 11
  rest and exercise, 11, 12, 14
Arthritis Foundation, 153

Arthritis and Parkinsonism
  body mechanics, 157
  Insert-a-Foot Shoe Aid, 157
  rheumatoid arthritis, 157
  self-help devices, 157
  Swedish reacher, 157
  wristlet, 157
Arthritis, rheumatoid, 11, *12*, 13, 128, 147, 148, 157
  ankylosis, 147
  deforming force, *12*, 147
  dislocation, 147
  joint disorders, 147
  joint inflammation, 147
  muscle weakness, 147
  osteoarthritis, *13*, 147
  pain, 147
  range of motion (ROM), 147
  subluxation, 147
  See also Arthritis; Osteoarthritis
Aspirin, 12, 13
Assistive devices, 32, 86, 87-88, 91
  braces, 87
  dropped foot, 87
  functional long leg, 88, 91
  knee immobilizers, 88
  lifts, 87
  See also Walking aids
Atherosclerosis, 3
Attention span, reduced, 112
  See also Aphasia
Austin-Moore prosthesis, 32
Axons, 3
  motor, 3

B

Balance training, 6
Basal ganglia, 10, 11
Bed activities, 30, 33
  bed positioning, 33, 37, 39
  moving sideways, 33, 59, 60
  moving up and down, 33, 58, 59
  range of motion (ROM), 33
  rolling over, 33, 61, 62
Bed bath, 38, 39
Bed pan exercises, 60
Bed rest, 17, 18, 20
  inactivity, 18
  negative effects of, 17, 20
Be OK Self-Help Aids, 131, 134, 141, 143, 144, 148, 149, 150, 160
Bladder training, 182, 183, 184, 185, 186, *187*, 188
  bacteremia, 185, 186
  catheter, 185, 186
  epididymitis, 185
  identification and management of bladder problems, 183
  incontinence, 186
  intake-output records, 186, 188
  nocturnal incontinence, 186, 188

pyelonephritis, 185
  record for training, 187
  voiding, 183, 184, 186
Blindness, 6
Body mechanics, 26, 27, 28, 29, 31, 62, 78, 84, 152, 157
  activities, 27
  basic principles, 26
  procedure for getting patient from bed, 27, 65
  safety points, 29
  See also Arthritis and Parkinsonism; Energy conservation and work simplification
Book butler, 143
  See also Reading
Book holder, 143
  See also Activities of daily living (ADL); Reading
Bowel, 9, 176, 177, 179, 180
  control, 9
  digital exam, 179, 180
  Fleets with oil, 178
  incontinence, 179, 180
  neurogenic, 176, 179
  problems, 176-177
  soap suds enema, 178
Brain, *3*, 7
  frontal cross section, *3*
Built-up handle, 131, 145, 149, 153, 157
  Spoon, 131, 145, 157
  See also Eating, self-help devices
Butazolidine, 13
Button hook, 151
  See also Self-care training

C

Canes, 100, 101, 104, 105, 107,
  quad canes, 100, 104, 105
Card holder, 144
  See also Activities of daily living (ADL)
Cardiac Symptoms, 20, 21
Card shuffler, automatic, 144
  See also Activities of daily living (ADL)
Catheter care, 187, 188
  Betadine, 187
  bulb-type catheter syringe, 188
  Foley urethral catheter, 187, 188
  Neosporin, 187
  perineal care, 187
  Toomey syringe, 188
  urinary tract infection, 187
Cartilage, *12*
Cerebral thrombosis, 5
Cerebral vascular accident, 7
Chamber of Commerce, 123
Clinical instruction, 207, 208, 209
  .clinical experience, 208
  evaluation, 209
  human element, 207, 208
  questioning techniques, 208
Communication book, 111
  See also dysarthria

Communication
    dysarthria, 113
    laryngectomy, 113
Communication impairments, 110, 111
Communication process, 111, 112
    aphasia, 112
    hearing impairments, 111
    input, 111
    output, 111
    speech impairment, 111
Communication techniques, basic, 112-113
Constipation, 176, 177, 178, 179, 180
    anorexia, 177, 180
    cramps, 177, 178, 180
    distension, 177, 180
    laxative, 177, 178
    prophylaxis, 177, 180
    table for management of, 178
Cortex, 3, 10
    motor, 10
    sensorimotor, 3
Corticosteroids, 12, 13
    intra-articular, 12, 13
    oral, 12
Crutches, 99, 103, 105
    gait, 99
Cut-out window, 144
    See also Reading

D

Dantrium, 5, 8, 11
Decubiti. See Pressure sores
Decussation, 3
    motor, 3
    sensory, 3
Denial, 119, 120, 121
    reality person, 120
    See also Emotional problems
Dentures and denture adhesive
    See Stroke
Department of Public Welfare, 123
Diabetes, 36
Diagnoses, 32
    accompanying disabilities, 32
    common, 32
Diarrhea, 176, 177
Disabilities. See Diagnoses
Disability-specific therapy, 7
Disability syndrome, 2
Discharge planning, 122-123
Dressing procedures or techniques, 135-143, 151,
    152, 155, 156
    bra, 139-140
    braces, 141
    button hook, 151
    buttoning and unbuttoning, 135
    clothespin, 151
    coat, 136
    dresses, 135

elastic shoe laces, 143
FashionABLE, 151
Insert-A-Foot Shoe Aid, 141
one-hand bow, 142
one-handed typing, 142
pants, 135, 138, 139
sequence for training, 135-143
shirt, 135-136, 145, 155-156
shoes, 141-142, 156
shorts, 138-139
skirts, 135
slip, 136-138
socks, 140, 151, 156
stockings, device to put on, 151-152
undershirt, 136-138
velcro closures, 141, 142, 155, 156
vocational guidance and rehabilitation services,
    151
Dysarthria, 111, 112, 113
    alphabet card, 111
    communication book, 111
    See also Aphasia; Communication; Speech im-
    pairment

E

Eating, 130-133, 145, 148-149
    interlace utensil holder, 149
    IV support, 130
    nasogastric tube, 130
    plate guard, 131
    self-help feeding devices, 130-133
    spoon with built-up handle, 131
    straw, 131
    suction cup, 131, 145
    suction holder, 131
    swallowing, 130
    washcloth, 131
Emboli, 4, 7
Embolic theory, 3
Embroidery, 144
    frame, 145
    See also Sewing
Emotional adjustments, 129, 130
Emotional lability, 112
    See also Aphasia
Emotional problems, 119, 120, 122, 124
    denial, 119, 124
    fear, 119, 124
    rejection, 120, 124
Energy conservation and work simplification,
    152-153
    body mechanics, 152
    Swedish reacher, 153
    See also Self-help devices
Esophageal speech. See Laryngectomy
Extensors, 4

F

FashionABLE, 131, 134, 143, 144, 149, 150, 151, 153, 160
Fatigue, 112
  See also Aphasia
Fear, 119, 121
  anxiety, 119, 121
  depression, 119, 121
  See also Emotional problems
Fertility, 9
  female, 9
  male, 9
Flexors, 4, 5, 39
  finger, 39
Footboards, 36
  See also Ankles, area to be positioned
Fractured hip, 32
  closed reduction, 32
  surgically pinned, 32

G

Gait, 11, 85-86, 91, 99, 100, 101, 106
  cane first, 100
  cane together, 101
  functional long leg, 86, 91
  normal gait, 85-86, 91
  shuffling, 11
  stance phase, 85
  step through pattern, 99, 100
  step-to pattern, 99, 101
  swing phase, 86
Gait training, 82-85
  am I ready, 82
  cardiac precautions, 83
  correct guarding, 83-84
  safest gait, 83
  shoes, good, 83
  test, 84
Gastrocenemius, 39
Gold salts, 12

H

Head, area to be positioned, 34
Hearing aids, 111
  See also Hearing impairment
Hearing impairment, 111
  hearing aids, 111
  presbycusis, 111
  speech reading, 111.
  See also Communication process
Hearing loss, 112, 113
Hemianopsia, 6, 7, 32, 112, 132-133, 144, 145, 163
  homonymous hemianopsia, 167
  See also Aphasia, Hemiplegia
Hemiplegia, 2, 3, 4, 5, 6, 7, 100, 128, 129, 130, 145, 146, 147, 148, 149, 215
  dressing techniques, 145

emotional adjustment, 129, 130
hemianopsia, 145
one-handed techniques, 129
self-care training, 129, 145
self-help devices, 145
sling, 129, 146
  See also Self-care training
Hemispheric specialization, 5
Hemorrhage, 3
Hirschberg, Dr. Gerard, 19
Home health agencies, 123, 124
  city health, 123, 124
  county health, 123, 124
  Visiting Nurses Association, 123
Homemaking and Work
  simplifications, 145
  American Heart Association, 145
  Mealtime Manual for the Aged and Handicapped, 145
  See also Activities of daily living

I

Incontinence, types of, 179, 180, 183, 184, 185, 186, 188
  Crede maneuver, 184
  high spinal cord dysfunction, 183, 185
  hydronephrosis, 184
  low spinal cord dysfunction, 184, 185
  mechanical urethral obstruction, 184
  pyelonephritis, 184, 185
  reverse flow (reflux), 184, 185, 186
  stress, 183, 185
  test, 184-185
  urge, 183, 185
  See also Bladder training; Bowel
Indomethecin, 12, 13
Infarction, 3, 7
  cerebral, 7
Insert-a-Foot Shoe Aid, 141, 157
  See also Arthritis and Parkinsonism; Dressing procedures or techniques
Intellectual loss, 9
Intercostals, 8
Interlace utensil holder, 149
  See also Eating; Self-help devices for eating
Internal capsule, 3, 11

J

Joints, 11, 32
  metacarpophalangeal, 11

K

Knees, area to be positioned, 34

L

Language symbols, 112
   See also Aphasia
Laryngeal dysfunction. *See* Voice problems
Laryngectomy, 111, 113
   esophageal speech, 111
   larynx, 111
   See also Communication
Larynx, 112
   See also Laryngectomy
Laxative, 177, 178, 179, 180
   Dulcolax, 178, 179
   Metamucil, 177, 180
   MOM, 177
   Senacott, 178, 180
   See also Constipation
L-dopa, 10, 11
Legs, area to be positioned, 35
Lesions, 7, 8, 9, 11
   complete, 8, 9
   fixed, 7
   high on spinal cord, 8
   partial, 8
   within the internal capsule, 7

M

Mealtime Manual for the Aged and Handicapped,
   145, 153
   See also Activities of daily living (ADL); Home-
   making and work simplifications
Medicare, 122
Medulla, 3
Memory impairment, 112
   See also Aphasia
Mirror, around the neck, 150
   See also Self-care devices for personal hygiene
Mobilization, 39
Motrin, 12
Movement, restoration of, 193, 194, 195, 196, 199
   ischial tuberosities, 193, 196, 199
   shifting weight, 194
   turning schedule, 195
   using siderails, 194
   wheelchair pushups, 194
Muscles, 11, 12
Myositis ossifications, 40

N

Neural transmission, 8
Neurochairs, 166
   See also Wheelchairs
Neurological return, spontaneous, 5
Neurons, 3, 5
No-tip glass keeper, 149
   See also Self-help devices for eating

O

One-hand bow, 142
   See also Dressing procedures or techniques
One-handed tying, 142
   See also Dressing procedures or techniques
Optic fibers, 6
Osteoarthritis, 12, 13, 147
   degenerative process, 147
   See Arthritis; Rheumatoid arthritis
Otolaryngologist
   See Voice problems

P

Paraplegic, 71, 163, 165, 171, 183, 184, 193, 200
Paresis, 4
Paretic hand, 5
Parkinsonism, 2, 10, 32, 34, 35, 128, 147, 153, 154, 155,
   156, 157
   activities of daily living (ADL), 156
   arthritis and Parkinsonism, 157
   body mechanics, 157
   Insert-A-Foot Shoe Aid, 157
   lack of automatic movement, 154
   rheumatoid arthritis, 157
   rigidity, 154, 155
   self-help devices, 155
   self-help devices for dressing procedures, 155
   self-help devices for eating, 155
   self-help devices for personal hygiene, 155
   Swedish reacher, 157
   tremor, 154, 155
   wristlet, 155
Participant observation, 209, 210, 211, 212
   diary of observations, 210, 211
   event, 210, 211, 212
   observer, 210, 211, 212
   place, 210, 211, 212
   time, 210, 211, 212
   See also Clinical instruction; Self-instructional
   materials
Peristalsis, 177, 179, 180
Personal hygiene procedures, 128, 133-134, 155
   antiperspirant, 133
   bathing, 134
   combing hair, 133
   dentures, 155
   denture toothbrush, one-handed, 134
   fingernail brush, one-handed, 134
   make-up, 133
   oral hygiene, 133
   self-help devices, 133-134
   shaving, toothpaste unscrewing, one-handed,
   133
   wristlet, 155
Phone amplifier, 144
   See also Telephone
Plate guard, 146
Plaque, 4

Pons, 3
Pregait training, 63, 64, 65, 66-70, 70-71, 71-73
   dizziness, 64, 65
   sitting balance, 65-66
   sitting position, 64-65
   transfers, 66-70
   trunk control, 66
   weight shifting, 71
   wheelchair ambulation, 70-71
   wheelchair exercise, 71-73
   See also Transfers; Wheelchair ambulation and
      weight shifting
Presbycusis, 111
   See also Hearing impairment
Pressure sores, 36, 37, 71, 72, 102, 193, 195, 196, 197,
   198, 199, 200, 201
   anemia, 200
   decubitus formation, 193, 200
   doughnuts, *196*
   edema, 200
   foam padding, *196*
   horsehoe-shaped cushions, *196*
   hyperemia, 193
   necrosis, 193, 200
   osteomyelitis, 200
   pillows, *196*
   prone position, 198
   seat boards, 197
   side lying, *198*
   sitting, *199*
   Spenko Stryker Boot, *196*
   supine position, *198*
   surface modifications, 195, 201
   surgery and/or grafting, 201
   tissue, normal and edematous, *199*
   turning frames, *197*
   water beds, 197
Pretest/posttest design, 209, 212
   See also Clinical instruction; Self-instructional
      materials
Progressive mobilization, 16, 17, 18, 19, 20, 21, 26, 29,
   30, 31, 32, 33, 37, 63, 79, 81, 82, 106, 207, 215
   staircase, 207
Progressive resistive exercises (PRE), 40
Prosthesis, total hip. *See* Austin-Moore prosthesis
Psycho-social aspects of patient and his family, 116,
   117, 119
   environmental resources, 117, 119
   financial resources, 117, 119
   personal resources, 117, 119
Psycho-social rehabilitation, 118
Pulse rate, 21, 22, 23, 25, 31, 205
   activity-related, 22, 23, 58, 60, 64, 74, 83
   how to take, 21, 22, 205
   monitoring, 21
   resting, 31
   rhythm, 22
Pulse response, 24
   sitting, 25

Q

Quadriplegic, 163, 170, 171, 183

R

Range of motion (ROM), 33, 36, 38, 147, 148, 149, 150,
   151, 153, 154, 155, 157
   abduction, 37
   active range of motion (ROM), 38, 58
   adduction, 37
   ankles, 39
   circumduction, 37
   dorsiflexion, 37
   exercises, 106
   extension, 37
   flexion, 37
   functional activities for range of motion (ROM),
      38, 58
   hemiplegic self-range of motion (ROM), *41, 42,
      43, 44, 45, 46, 47, 48, 49, 50*
   passive range of motion (ROM), 38, 40, 41, 58
   plantar flexion, 37
   pronation, 37
   range of motion by nurse, *41, 42, 43, 44, 45, 46, 47,
      48, 49, 50-57*
   supination, 37
   test for, 40
Reading, 143-144
   book butler, 143
   book holder, 143
   cut-out window, 144
   See also Activities of daily living
Reality person, *120*
   See also Denial
Reflexes, 5, 7
   uninhibited stretch, 7
Rehabilitation, 7, 38, 116, 158, 215
   physical, 215
   self-help devices, 158
   street clothes, 158
   techniques, 7
Rejection, 120, 121
   education, 120
   encouragement, 120
   See also Emotional problems
Respiratory problems, 8
Retina, blind, *6*
Rheumatoid arthritis, 147-148
   joint disorders, 147
   muscle weakness, 147
   pain, 147
   range of motion, 147
Rigidity, 10, 11
Rocker knife, 146
   See also Self-help devices for eating

S

Self-care training, 128, 129, 130, 145, 148-149, 153, 154-155, 158
  activities of daily living (ADL), 148
  hemiplegia, 148
  range of motion (ROM), 148, 149
  self-care devices, 128, 129, 148, 157
  See also Self-help devices
Self-help devices, 146, 147, 148-153, 154, 155, 157, 158
  See Arthritis and Parkinsonism; Rehabilitation; Self-care training
Self-help devices for eating, 146, 148, 155
  built-up handle, 149
  interlace utensil holder, 149
  no-tip glass keeper, 149
  range of motion (ROM), 148
  rocker knife, 146
  straw holder, 149
  swivel spoon, 149
  universal cuff or utensil holder, 149
  wristlet, 149
  wrist splint, 149
Self-help devices for personal hygiene, 149-151
  arthritis, 149
  bathing, 150
  button hook, 151
  combing hair, 150
  dressing, 151-152
  fingernails, 150
  hemiplegia, 149
  long-handled comb and brush, 150
  make-up, 149-150
  mirror, around the neck, 150
  oral hygiene, 150
  range of motion (ROM), 149
  razor, manual, 149
  shaving, 149
  shoehorn, long, 152
  stockings, device to put on, 152
  Swedish reacher, 153
  Velcro, 151
Self-instructional materials, 204, 205, 206, 209, 212
  evaluation, 209
  feedback loops, 205, 206
  objectives, 205
  self-paced, 205, 206
Sensors (muscle spindles), 5
Sensory loss, 5
Sewing, 144
  embroidery, 144
  embroidery frame, 144
  See also Activities of daily living (ADL)
Sex, 9
  sexual function, 9
Sinemet, 10
Sitting, 23, 24, 30
  tolerance schedule, 24, 30, 65, 66
Sling, 129, 146

Slow learning, 130
Social Security Office, 123, 124
Social services, 123
Spasticity, 5, 7, 9, 11
Speech impairment, 111, 112
  aphasia, 112
  dysarthria, 111
  laryngectomy, 111
  voice problems, 111
  See also Communication process
Speech pathologist, 110
Speech reading, 111
  See also Hearing impairment
Spinal cord, 2, 8, 9
  disability syndrome, *8*
  dysfunction, 8, 9
Staircase, *18, 19*, 30, 32, 33
  bed activities, 32
  dependent, *18, 19*
  independent, *18, 19,* 30, 33
  sitting, 32
  stair/climbing, 32
  standing, 32
  transfers, 32
  walking, 32
Stairclimbing, 76-79, 80
  crutch-railing method, *79*
  going up and going down, *78*
  methods using crutches, 79
  two-crutch method, going up and going down, *79*
Standing, 73-76, 80
  standing balance, 75-76
  stand-ups, 73-75, 76
State Department of Public Welfare, 123, 124
Stockings, device to put on, 152
  See also Dressing procedures or techniques; Self-care devices for personal hygiene
Stool, 177, 178, 179, 180
Straw holder, 149
  See also Eating
Stress, 25
Stroke, 32, 35, 111, 143, 146, 183, 210
  dentures and denture adhesive, 111
  See also Incontinence; Hemiplegia
Subdural hematoma, 3
Subluxation, 11, *12,* 129, 147
  See also Rheumatoid Arthritis
Swedish reacher, 153, 157
  See also Arthritis and Parkinsonism; Energy conservation and work simplification; Self-care devices
Swivel spoon, 149, 153
  See also Self-help devices for eating
Syncope, 24
Synovium, 11, *12*

T

Telephone, 144
  amplifier, 144
  See also Activities of daily living

Tendon, *12*
Thrombi, 7
Tracheostomy. *See* Voice problems
Transfers, 66-70, 73
  sliding board, 69-70
  standing, 67-68
Transient ischemic attacks (TIAS), 3
Tremor, 10, 11
  hand tremor, 11
  pill rolling 10
Trunk stability, 9
Tumor, 3
  benign, 3
  malignant primary, 3
  metastatic, 3

U

United Fund Division-Community Chest, 123
Utensil, 148-149, 153, 157
  holder, 149, 153
  long-handled, 153, 157
  universal cuff, 149
  See also Eating, Self-help devices for eating

V

Valium, 8, 11
Vasodilators, 7
Velcro, 141, 142-143, 151, 155, 156
  See also Dressing procedures or techniques;
    Parkinsonism; Self-care training
Verticality perception, 6
Vertigo, 10
Visual field, *6*
  blind portion of, *6*
Visual loss, 112
Vitamins, 7, 10, 11
  B6, 10, 11
  B12, 7
Vocal cords. *See* Voice problems
Vocational guidance of rehabilitation service, 160
Voice problems, 111
  laryngeal dysfunction, 111
  otolaryngologist, 111
  tracheostomy, 111
Vocal cords, 111
  See also Speech impairment

W

Walker, 103, 105, 106, 163
Walkcane, 89, 92, 100, 101, 105, 107
Walking aids, 36, 88-105
  cane, 94
  crutches, 36, 89, 91, 92, 93, 96-100
  measuring aids—five rules, 93, 94
  turning around, 102
  standing a patient from a chair, 91-92
  walkers, 36, 88, 89, 91, 93, 95

Walking step, 30
Wheelchairs, 44, 45, 102-103, 106, 162-173
  backing up and sitting down, 102-103, 106
  maintenance, 172-173
  neurochair, 166
  standard dimensions, *164*
  wheelchair parts, 69, 164-171
Wheelchair ambulation and weight shifting, 70-72, 80
  modified push-up, 71
  moving a wheelchair patient, *72*
  pulling, 71
  wheelchair exercise, 71
  wheelchair push-ups, 71
Wristlet, 149, 155, 157
  See also Arthritis and Parkinsonism; Parkin-
    sonism; Personal hygiene procedures; Self-
    help devices for eating
Writing, 144
  clipboard, 144
  prewriting exercises, 144
  writing examples, 144
  See also Activities of daily living (ADL)
Wrist splint, 49
  See also Self-help devices for eating